T0263306

Human Factors and Technology in the ICU

Editor

SHU-FEN WUNG

CRITICAL CARE NURSING CLINICS OF NORTH AMERICA

www.ccnursing.theclinics.com

Consulting Editor
JAN FOSTER

June 2018 • Volume 30 • Number 2

ELSEVIER

1600 John F. Kennedy Boulevard • Suite 1800 • Philadelphia, Pennsylvania, 19103-2899

http://www.theclinics.com

CRITICAL CARE NURSING CLINICS OF NORTH AMERICA Volume 30, Number 2
June 2018 ISSN 0899-5885, ISBN-13: 978-0-323-58395-4

Editor: Kerry Holland
Developmental Editor: Laura Fisher

© **2018 Elsevier Inc. All rights reserved.**

This periodical and the individual contributions contained in it are protected under copyright by Elsevier, and the following terms and conditions apply to their use:

Photocopying
Single photocopies of single articles may be made for personal use as allowed by national copyright laws. Permission of the Publisher and payment of a fee is required for all other photocopying, including multiple or systematic copying, copying for advertising or promotional purposes, resale, and all forms of document delivery. Special rates are available for educational institutions that wish to make photocopies for non-profit educational classroom use. For information on how to seek permission visit www.elsevier.com/permissions or call: (+44) 1865 843830 (UK)/(+1) 215 239 3804 (USA).

Derivative Works
Subscribers may reproduce tables of contents or prepare lists of articles including abstracts for internal circulation within their institutions. Permission of the Publisher is required for resale or distribution outside the institution. Permission of the Publisher is required for all other derivative works, including compilations and translations (please consult www.elsevier.com/permissions).

Electronic Storage or Usage
Permission of the Publisher is required to store or use electronically any material contained in this periodical, including any article or part of an article (please consult www.elsevier.com/permissions). Except as outlined above, no part of this publication may be reproduced, stored in a retrieval system or transmitted in any form or by any means, electronic, mechanical, photocopying, recording or otherwise, without prior written permission of the Publisher.

Notice
No responsibility is assumed by the Publisher for any injury and/or damage to persons or property as a matter of products liability, negligence or otherwise, or from any use or operation of any methods, products, instructions or ideas contained in the material herein. Because of rapid advances in the medical sciences, in particular, independent verification of diagnoses and drug dosages should be made.

Although all advertising material is expected to conform to ethical (medical) standards, inclusion in this publication does not constitute a guarantee or endorsement of the quality or value of such product or of the claims made of it by its manufacturer.

Critical Care Nursing Clinics of North America (ISSN 0899-5885) is published quarterly by Elsevier Inc., 360 Park Avenue South, New York, NY 10010-1710. Months of issue are March, June, September, and December. Business and Editorial Offices: 1600 John F. Kennedy Blvd., Suite 1800, Philadelphia, PA 19103-2899. Periodicals postage paid at New York, NY and additional mailing offices. Subscription prices are $155.00 per year for US individuals, $385.00 per year for US institutions, $100.00 per year for US students and residents, $200.00 per year for Canadian individuals, $483.00 per year for Canadian institutions, $230.00 per year for international individuals, $483.00 per year for international institutions and $115.00 per year for Canadian and international students/residents. To receive student/resident rate, orders must be accompanied by name of affiliated institution, data of term, and the *signature* of program/residency coordinator on institution letterhead. Orders will be billed at individual rate until proof of status is received. Foreign air speed delivery is included in all *Clinics* subscription prices. All prices are subject to change without notice. **POSTMASTER:** Send address changes to *Critical Care Nursing Clinics of North America*, Elsevier Health Sciences Division, Subscription Customer Service, 3251 Riverport Lane, Maryland Heights, MO 63043. **Customer Service: 1-800-654-2452 (US and Canada); 314-447-8871 (outside US and Canada). Fax: 314-447-8029. E-mail:** JournalsCustomerService-usa@elsevier.com **(for print support) and** JournalsOnlineSupport-usa@elsevier.com **(for online support).**

Reprints. For copies of 100 or more of articles in this publication, please contact the Commercial Reprints Department, Elsevier Inc., 360 Park Avenue South, New York, New York, 10010-1710; Tel.: 212-633-3874, Fax: 212-633-3820, and E-mail: reprints@elsevier.com.

Critical Care Nursing Clinics of North America is covered in *MEDLINE/PubMed (Index Medicus), International Nursing Index, Nursing Citation Index, Cumulative Index to Nursing and Allied Health Literature, and RNdex Top 100.*

Contributors

CONSULTING EDITOR

JAN FOSTER, PhD, APRN, CNS
Formerly, Associate Professor, College of Nursing, Texas Woman's University, Houston, Texas, USA; Currently, President, Nursing Inquiry and Intervention, Inc, The Woodlands, Texas, USA

EDITOR

SHU-FEN WUNG, PhD, RN, ACNP-BC, FAAN
Associate Professor, Biobehavioral Health Science Division, The University of Arizona College of Nursing, Tucson, Arizona, USA

AUTHORS

SOPHIA AIRHART, MD
The University of Arizona College of Medicine, Sarver Heart Center, Tucson, Arizona, USA

RUTH A. ANDERSON, PhD, RN, FAAN
School of Nursing, The University of North Carolina at Chapel Hill, Chapel Hill, North Carolina, USA

WILLIAM J. BINDER, PharmD
The University of Arizona College of Medicine, Tucson, Arizona, USA

RUSSELL J. BRANAGHAN, PhD
Human Systems Engineering Program, Ira A. Fulton Schools of Engineering, Arizona State University, Mesa, Arizona, USA

BARBARA B. BREWER, PhD, RN, MALS, MBA, FAAN
The University of Arizona College of Nursing, Tucson, Arizona, USA

JAMES FORREST CALLAND, MD
School of Medicine, University of Virginia, Charlottesville, Virginia, USA

PASCALE CARAYON, PhD
Professor, Department of Industrial and Systems Engineering, Director, Center for Quality and Productivity Improvement, University of Wisconsin-Madison, Madison, Wisconsin, USA

JANE M. CARRINGTON, PhD, RN, FAAN
The University of Arizona College of Nursing, Tucson, Arizona, USA

MATTHEW T. CLARK, PhD
Advanced Medical Predictive Devices, Diagnostics and Displays, Inc, Charlottesville, Virginia, USA

JENNIFER L. COOK, MD
The University of Arizona College of Medicine, Tucson, Arizona, USA

LINDA FAHEY, DNP, MSN
Chief Operating Officer and Senior Vice President of Quality Systems Administration, Decatur Memorial Hospital, Decatur, Illinois, USA

DAN FRACZKOWSKI, MSN, RN
Clinical Nursing Consultant, Information Services, University of Illinois Hospital & Health Sciences System, Chicago, Illinois, USA

MARJORIE FUNK, PhD, RN, FAHA, FAAN
Helen Porter Jayne and Martha Prosser Jayne Professor of Nursing, Yale School of Nursing, West Haven, Connecticut, USA

KAREN K. GIULIANO, PhD, RN, FAAN, MBA
Associate Professor of Nursing, Northeastern University, External Faculty Nurse Scientist, Yvonne L. Munn Center for Nursing Research, Massachusetts General Hospital, Boston, Massachusetts, USA; Nurse Scientist, Center for Nursing Research and Advanced Practice, Orlando Health, Orlando, Florida, USA

NICKALAUS GRAMZE, MD
Banner-University Medical Center Phoenix, Phoenix, Arizona, USA

PETER L.T. HOONAKKER, PhD
Senior Scientist, Center for Quality and Productivity Improvement, University of Wisconsin-Madison, Madison, Wisconsin, USA

JESSICA KEIM-MALPASS, PhD, RN
Assistant Professor, School of Nursing, School of Medicine, University of Virginia, Charlottesville, Virginia, USA

REBECCA R. KITZMILLER, PhD, MHR, RN, BC
School of Nursing, The University of North Carolina at Chapel Hill, Chapel Hill, North Carolina, USA

CURT LINDBERG, DMan
Billings Clinic, Billings, Montana, USA

KAREN DUNN LOPEZ, PhD, MPH, RN
Assistant Professor, Health Systems Science, University of Illinois at Chicago College of Nursing, Chicago, Illinois, USA

DANIEL C. MALONE, RPh, PhD
Professor, The University of Arizona College of Pharmacy, Tucson, Arizona, USA

J. RANDALL MOORMAN, MD
School of Medicine, University of Virginia, Advanced Medical Predictive Devices, Diagnostics and Displays, Inc, Charlottesville, Virginia, USA

CHRISTINE W. NIBBELINK, PhD, RN
Department of Biomedical Informatics, University of California, San Diego, La Jolla, California, USA

ARIANI ARISTA PUTRI PERTIWI, DNP, MSN, RN
Department of Basic Nursing and Emergency, Faculty of Medicine, Lecturer, Universitas Gadjah Mada, JI, PSIK, FK, Yogyakarta, Indonesia

HALLEY RUPPEL, MS, RN
PhD Candidate, Robert Wood Johnson Foundation Future of Nursing Scholar,
Yale School of Nursing, West Haven, Connecticut, USA

MARILYN ROSE SCHATZ, DNP, RN, ACNP-BC
Nurse Practitioner, Pulmonary Consultants of Mesa, Mesa, Arizona, USA

ANGELA SKEELES-WORLEY, MEd
School of Education, University of Virginia, Charlottesville, Virginia, USA

SHERYL L. STOGIS, DrPH, RN
Assistant Clinical Professor, College of Nursing, University of Illinois at Chicago, Chicago,
Illinois, USA

KEVIN SULLIVAN, PhD
School of Engineering, University of Virginia, Charlottesville, Virginia, USA

LAURA SZALACHA, EdD
Professor, Director of Research Methods and Statistics, The University of Arizona College
of Nursing, Tucson, Arizona, USA

ROBERT TAI, EdD
School of Education, University of Virginia, Charlottesville, Virginia, USA

SHU-FEN WUNG, PhD, RN, ACNP-BC, FAAN
Associate Professor, Biobehavioral Health Science Division, The University of Arizona
College of Nursing, Tucson, Arizona, USA

JANAY R. YOUNG, DNP, RN
Special Immunology Associates, El Rio Community Health Center, The University of
Arizona College of Nursing, Tucson, Arizona, USA

Contents

> In this focus group study, we identified issues associated with sensory over-load from medical technology alarms or alerts for intensive care unit nurses. Participants indicated that alarms from cardiopulmonary monitors, ventilators, and intravenous pumps contributed the most to sensory overload and, yet, these alarms were also deemed the most helpful. Alerts or alarms from electronic health records and medication dispensing systems were rated low in contributing to sensory overload, as well as being the least helpful. Specific device or technology barriers, related to device alerts or alarms, are detailed. Future user-centered and integrated improvements in alarm systems associated with medical devices in the intensive care unit are needed.

> This study uniquely gained insight into the intricacy of intensive care nurses' decision-making process when responding to and managing device alarms. Difficulty in responding to alarms included low staffing, multiple job responsibilities, and competing priority tasks. Novice nurses are more tolerant of alarms sounding owing to a lower threshold of comfort with resetting or silencing alarms; more experienced nurses are more comfortable resetting alarm limits to the patient's baseline. Understanding the decision-making process used by nurses can guide the development of policies and learning experiences that are crucial clinical support for alarm management.

> Nurses are the end users of most technology in intensive care units, and the ways in which they interact with technology affect quality of care and patient safety. Nurses' interactions include the processes of ensuring proper input of data into the technology as well as extracting and interpreting the output (clinical data, technical data, alarms). Current challenges in nurse-technology interactions for physiologic monitoring include issues regarding alarm management, workflow interruptions, and monitor surveillance. Patient safety concepts, such as high reliability organizations and human factors, can advance efforts to enhance nurse-technology interactions.

> With an estimated 90% of all hospitalized patients receiving intravenous medications via infusion pumps, intravenous infusion pump systems are

among the most frequently used technologies in health care. This article reviews important issues regarding clinical usability, intravenous medication administration error, and patient safety related to the use of intravenous smart pumps. Although it is possible to address some of the issues with changes in clinical processes, the most fundamental challenges need to be addressed through innovation and the development of new technologies using a human factors approach.

About 400,000 to 500,000 patients die in intensive care units (ICUs) each year, largely because ICUs care for the sickest patients. On the other hand, factors such as workload, shift changes, handoffs, alarm fatigue, inadequate team communication, and difficult-to-use medical devices contribute to the problem. This article focuses on the human factors of those medical devices, a significant cause of adverse events in the ICU.

Critical care nurses practice in a challenging environment that requires responses to patients with complex, often unstable health conditions. The electronic health record, access to clinical data, and Clinical Decision Support Systems informed by data from clinical databases are informatics tools designed to work together to facilitate decision-making in nursing practice. The complex decision-making environment of critical care requires informatics tools that support nursing practice through integration of current evidence with clinical data. Recommendations include continuing efforts toward the development of clinical decision support tools based on patient data that include predictive models to support increased patient safety.

Health care, especially intensive care units, relies on multiple types of technology to promote the best patient outcomes. Unfortunately, too often these technologies are poorly designed, causing errors, additional workload, and unnecessary frustration. This article (1) empowers nurses with the needed usability and usability testing vocabulary to identify and articulate clinical technology usability problems and (2) provides ideas on ways nurses can advocate to have an impact on positive change related to technology usability within a health care organization.

Tele-intensive care units (ICUs) are an innovation to handle issues such as personnel shortage and improving care. In tele-ICUs, clinical teams monitor ICU patients remotely and support clinicians in multiple ICUs. The tele-ICU and ICU clinicians function as virtual teams. Little is known how these teams function and what challenges they encounter. The authors examined the challenges from the perspective of nurses in a tele-ICU. They used a case study design and conducted interviews with 10 tele-ICU nurses. The nurses encounter challenges in interacting with the multiple ICUs that they monitor remotely and have developed strategies to cope with these challenges.

In the intensive care unit, clinicians monitor a diverse array of data inputs to detect early signs of impending clinical demise or improvement. Continuous predictive analytics monitoring synthesizes data from a variety of inputs into a risk estimate that clinicians can observe in a streaming environment. For this to be useful, clinicians must engage with the data in a way that makes sense for their clinical workflow in the context of a learning health system (LHS). This article describes the processes needed to evoke clinical action after initiation of continuous predictive analytics monitoring in an LHS.

Health systems across the United States are adopting intensive care unit telemedicine programs to improve patient outcomes. Research demonstrates the potential for decreased mortality and length of stay for patients of these remotely monitored units. Financial models and studies point to cost-effectiveness and the possibility of cost savings in the face of abundant startup costs. Questions remain as to the true financial implications of these programs and targeted populations that may see the greatest benefit. Despite recent growth, widespread adoption may be limited until these unknowns are answered.

Sepsis, life-threatening organ dysfunction in response to infection, is an alarmingly common and aggressive illness in US hospitals, especially for intensive care patients. Preventing sepsis deaths rests on the clinicians' ability to promptly recognize and treat sepsis. To aid early recognition, many organizations have employed clinician-facing electronic sepsis alert systems. However, the effectiveness of the alert relies heavily on the visual interface, textual information, and overall usability. This article reports a usability inspection of a sepsis alert system. The authors found violations in 12 of the 14 usability principles and promote use of this method in practice to systematically identify usability problems.

x

Human Factors and Technology in the ICU

CRITICAL CARE NURSING
CLINICS OF NORTH AMERICA

ISSUE OF RELATED INTEREST

Nursing Clinics, June 2015 (Vol. 50, Issue 2)
How Nursing has Changed with Technology
Francisca Cisneros Farrar, *Editor*
Available at: http://nursing.theclinics.com

THE CLINICS ARE AVAILABLE ONLINE!
Access your subscription at:
www.theclinics.com

Preface

Human Factors and Technology in the ICU

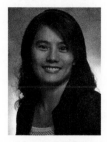

Shu-Fen Wung, PhD, RN, ACNP-BC, FAAN
Editor

Intensive care units (ICUs) are equipped with a multitude of technology to support the care of acutely ill patients with complex medical needs. The demanding nature of critical care nurses' work relies heavily on advanced health care technology as it has freed nurses from labor-intensive activities. In turn, nurses are expected to assume the role of expert in the use of health care technology. Yet, critical care nurses have identified insufficient and malfunctioning technology to be intensely stressful and threatening.[1]

Unlike other safety-critical industries, human factors research in health care, especially in nursing, under actual practice is long overdue. Traditionally, there is a greater emphasis on the technology itself than on nurse-technology interface. Such interface is essential as the less time nurses spend "nursing the machine," the more time they have available for direct patient care and the less dehumanizing the environment becomes.[2] The scientific field of human factors focuses on human strengths and limitations and the interaction between people, machines, and their work environment.[3] There is a major interest in the safety of medical devices/health technology by several organizations, including the US Food and Drug Administration, ECRI Institute, and others, and interactions between users and devices (the focus of human factors/usability engineering) is identified as the critical element.[4]

This special issue brings together 11 articles of diverse research and reviews regarding selected technology and critical care nurses' real-world experience interacting with these health care devices/technology in the ICU. Human factors/usability principles and issues are discussed to increase the awareness of the role of human factors for patient safety. Focusing on instruction or training fixes in isolation to mitigate user-technology hazards may improve safe and effective use of technology, but this is inadequate. Additional improvements to the technology and user-technology

Crit Care Nurs Clin N Am 30 (2018) xi–xii
https://doi.org/10.1016/j.cnc.2018.03.001
0899-5885/18/© 2018 Elsevier Inc. All rights reserved.

ccnursing.theclinics.com

interface by incorporating human factors considerations are critical for a safer ICU environment for patients and critical care nurses.

I would like to thank Dr. Jan Foster for inviting me to edit this important special topic for critical care nurses and for her full support.

Shu-Fen Wung, PhD, RN, ACNP-BC, FAAN
Biobehavioral Health Science Division
The University of Arizona College of Nursing
1305 N Martin Avenue
Tucson, AZ 85721-0203, USA

E-mail address:
wung@arizona.edu

REFERENCES

1. Sawatzky JA. Stress in critical care nurses: actual and perceived. Heart Lung 1996;25(5):409–17.
2. Hughes RG. Nurses at the "sharp end" of patient care. In: Hughes RG, editor. Patient safety and quality: an evidence-based handbook for nurses. Rockville (MD): Agency for Healthcare Research and Quality; 2008. p. 7–36.
3. Henrikson KDE, Keyes MA, Carayon P, et al. Chapter 5. Understanding adverse events: a human factor framework. In: Hughes RG, editor. Patient Safety and Quality: An Evidence-Based Handbook for Nurses, Vol 1. Rockville (MD): Agency for Healthcare Research and Quality; 2008. p. 1–21.
4. Human Factors and Medical Devices. Available at: https://www.fda.gov/Medical Devices/DeviceRegulationandGuidance/HumanFactors/default.htm. Accessed January 22, 2018.

Sensory Overload and Technology in Critical Care

Shu-Fen Wung, PhD, RN, ACNP-BC[a],*, Daniel C. Malone, RPh, PhD[b], Laura Szalacha, EdD[a]

KEYWORDS

- Sensory overload • Technology • Device alarms • Intensive care • Human factors

KEY POINTS

- Critical care nurses identified alarms from cardiopulmonary physiologic monitors, ventilators, and IV pumps as contributing most to sensory overload and as the most helpful ones.
- Barriers of cardiopulmonary physiologic monitor alerts/alarms include being unable to silence alarms, difficulty adjusting alarms, unable to recognize nontextbook rhythms, unable to recognize baseline rhythms, and being too sensitive.
- IV pump alarms were helpful for critical care nurses to know the array of IV drips administered were properly running.
- Barriers with IV pump alarms include unnecessary alarms while trouble-shooting, being overly sensitive, silence function with too short of duration, and loud and obnoxious alarm sounds.
- Several device/technology alarms make identical or nearly identical sounds regardless of their priority.

INTRODUCTION

The intensive care unit (ICU) has been characterized as a demanding work environment where the background noise of monitors, ventilators, and alarms and flashing lights are continuous.[1] In addition, the prompt attention required to continually turn off false alarms and monitor multiple devices for multiple patients is deemed often beyond the capabilities of most humans.[1] This high-stress environment is demanding physically, emotionally, and cognitively. As a result, critical care nurse burnout is pervasive and is the major reason nurses leave these intensive environments.[2–4] One-third of ICU nurses experience severe burnout and 60% of those with severe

Disclosure Statement: There is no commercial or financial conflicts of interest for all authors. There is no grant or other financial support used for the study.
[a] Biobehavioral Health Science Division, The University of Arizona College of Nursing, 1305 North Martin Avenue, Tucson, AZ 85721-0203, USA; [b] Pharmacy Practice and Science, The University of Arizona College of Pharmacy, 1295 North Martin Avenue, Tucson, AZ 85721-0202, USA
* Corresponding author.
E-mail address: wung@arizona.edu

burnout contemplated leaving the nursing profession.[5] Nurses often work 12-hour shifts, so it is not surprising that ICU nurses have the second highest turnover rates, second only to psychiatric units.[6]

Critically ill patients in the ICU are connected to an increasing number of monitors and life-sustaining medical devices. Managing the ever-evolving, sophisticated technology in the ICU is an expected skill for critical care nurses. Yet, critical care nurses have identified insufficient training and malfunctioning advanced technology to be stressful and threatening.[7] Moreover, noise levels in the ICUs often exceed recommended thresholds.[8] Critical care nurses report feeling fatigued, exasperated, and angry[9] from the constant bombardment of noise. Prolonged exposure to such noise often results in noise-induced stress, a predictor of burnout in critical care nurses.[10,11] Research has shown that people adapt to noisy work environments by becoming less interpersonally engaged, less caring, and less reflective.[8] Noise impedes the performance of complex intellectual tasks that require focused attention[12] and increases the frequency of errors in work environments.[13] Such negative performance effects from noise is more pronounced in those who are already experiencing sensory overload, defined as the state or condition produced by "overstimulation of one or more of the senses," and are working at near-capacity levels.[14] Therefore, improving the physical work environment of ICU is imperative.

A national survey of 6312 registered nurses from across Canada in 2010[15] reported that, "Fatigue has had its impact on nurses with 25.8% considering resigning; 20.2% considering retiring; and 25.6% considering leaving the profession owing to fatigue. ....Nurses also identified a feeling of sensory overload, functionally disorganized workplaces and relentless change within the workplace as contributors to their fatigue."[15] The purpose of this study was to identify issues and concerns associated with sensory overload among ICU nurses that are specifically related to medical device/technology generated alarms/alerts.

METHODS
Study Design

A qualitative study was conducted using focus groups with critical care nurses (working ≥20 hours per week over the past 6 months in a critical care environment). Participants for this study were identified through established contacts, emails, and study recruitment advertisements placed in critical care units. Critical care nurses with supervisory roles were excluded to avoid any concerns about participating from potential subjects. At beginning of each focus group, time was allotted to review the purpose of the study, answer questions, and obtain informed consent. The University of Arizona Human Subjects Protection Program reviewed and approved this project.

Pre–focus Group Survey

A preinterview survey was developed and completed before the structured interview. This self-administered questionnaire included (1) questions concerning demographic characteristics (participant age, gender, years in practice, years in critical care practice, and education), (2) asked participants to rate specific device alarms/alerts that contribute to sensory overload at work, and (3) asked participants to rate specific device alarms/alerts that are most helpful at work. These devices alarms/alerts included cardiopulmonary physiologic monitor auditory and visual alarms, nurse call light alarms, bed exit alarms, intravenous (IV) pump alarms, ventilator alarms, electronic health record (EHR) visual alerts, and medication dispensing systems. The participants rated each alert/alarm on a 10-point scale where 0 was contributing least to sensory overload or least helpful and 10 was contributing most to sensory overload or most helpful. Participants were encouraged to identify specific devices or alarms/alerts that they believed contributed to sensory overload and also were asked to comment on helpfulness of such alarms/alerts.

Each focus group was conducted over approximately 2 hours and was audio recorded and transcribed. Only the individual's first name was used during the focus group. The sessions addressed types and numbers of alarms/alerts (both visual and auditory) that require attention in the ICU, helpful and unhelpful alarms/alerts, ways to deal with annoying alerts/alerts help to achieve patient care goals, distractions and ways to minimize distractions, important tasks not wanted to be bothered by alerts, received and preferred trainings on responding to alerts/alarms, effects of alerts/alarms after work, alerts/alarms affecting patient outcomes, and alerts/alarms design improvement to reduce sensory overload. In this article, we examine helpful and unhelpful alarms/alerts experienced by critical care nurses and device/technology barriers specifically related to device alerts/alarms that contribute to sensory overload in the work setting. The questions asked included: "Can you provide examples of helpful and unhelpful auditory alarms/alerts? Why?" and "How could we design or improve alerts/alarms to reduce sensory overload?"

Data Analysis

Demographic data and ratings of specific device alarms/alerts that contribute to sensory overload as well as helpfulness of these device alarms/alerts were analyzed using descriptive statistics. All study investigators read and categorized the focus group data using a thematic topic coding approach. Topical coding included a general categorization followed by recoding to incorporate subcategories that were more specific. We identified types of auditory and visual alarms/alerts encountered, emotional responses to these alerts/alarms at work and after work, patient safety concerns, barriers and strategies used by critical care nurses to deal with alarms/alerts, and recommendations for technology improvement for alarms/alerts management to decrease sensory overload. Owing to the extensiveness of data collected, the focus of this article is on 2 major topics: helpful and unhelpful alarms/alerts experienced by critical care nurses and device/technology barriers, specifically related to device alerts/alarms that contribute to sensory overload in the work setting.

RESULTS
Participants

A total of 7 critical care nurses volunteered to participate in this study. All nurses were white women with a mean age of 29.1 ± 2.1 years. The average nursing and ICU experience was 3.4 ± 2.0 and 2.6 ± 1.6 years, respectively. The average weekly ICU work hours among these nurses was 37.1 ± 2.0. The majority of nurses (86%) had an undergraduate degree in nursing. The practice settings included trauma/neuro/surgical ICU (n = 2), cardiovascular ICU (n = 2), medical ICU (n = 2), and unspecified (n = 1).

Pre–focus Group Survey

Among 10 common device alerts/alarms, critical care nurses identified alarms from cardiopulmonary physiologic monitor, ventilator, and IV pump as contributing most to sensory overload, and yet these alarms were also deemed most helpful ones at work (**Table 1**). Alerts/alarms from EHR and medication dispensing system were rated low in contributing to sensory overload and the least helpful. Participants also added that bathroom call light alarms, tube feeding pump alarms, overhead paging, and

Table 1
Alerts/alarms contribute to sensory overload and helpfulness of these alerts/alarms

Alerts/Alarms	Contribute to Sensory Overload (Mean ± SD)	Helpfulness (Mean ± SD)
Cardiac monitor auditory	7.4 ± 0.8	6.3 ± 1.3
Ventilator	6.6 ± 1.7	7.0 ± 2.0
IV pump	6.0 ± 2.0	7.0 ± 1.6
Call light	5.9 ± 1.9	4.9 ± 1.6
Cardiac monitor visual	4.4 ± 1.9	6.6 ± 2.3
Bed exit	3.9 ± 3.0	6.0 ± 1.8
Electronic medical record	2.9 ± 2.1	3.1 ± 1.5
Medication dispensing system	2.6 ± 1.1	2.9 ± 1.5

Abbreviations: IV, intravenous; SE, standard deviation.

nurse phone were contributors to sensory overload. Alarms/alerts from specialty devices, including continuous renal replacement therapies, intraaortic balloon pump, extracorporeal membrane oxygenation, and left ventricular assist device/total artificial heart, were considered most helpful.

Types of Overwhelming Alerts/Alarms Encountered in the Intensive Care Unit

The critical care nurses encountered enormous numbers and types of alarms and these alarms came from many different devices that were not coordinated. "In the cardiac ICU…we have a whole variety of different devices… Each device has its own sound. Each alarm is totally different. It means something different. Gosh. There's probably 30 different kinds of alarms." Each alarm has a different, if not vitally important, function, "There's alarms for every little thing, every different rhythms. There's yellow alarms. There's red alarms." There isn't a hierarchy of these many alarms, "Everybody [every manufacturer] thinks their alarm is the most important alarm. I don't think they actually work in the unit and understand how many there are - the expert about this machine versus the expert on this machine." Alarms associated with multitude of medical devices/technologies in the ICU contributed to heightened sensory overload, "You're already gonna be stressed, because ICU is always stressful… When you have a to-do list this long, and you have a patient that's crashing, and you can't think about what you need to do, because you have these constant alarms that can just set you over the edge." Sensory overload from these alarms can affect the physical and mental health of critical care nurses, "It definitely tires you out. At the end of the day, being mentally tired … it's much more than being physically tired. Stimulated constantly for 12 hours." Alarms add to workload of critical care nurses, "They're [families] panicked that something's going on, that's something's really bad happening. Then on the other hand, then they might think negatively of you if it keeps alarming, and you ignore it. Yeah. Okay. If it's important enough to be alarming, and you're in the ICU, why aren't you paying attention to this?"

Auditory Alerts/Alarms

Participants identified several major monitoring and treatment devices that produce auditory alarms in the ICU. These include a ventilator, extracorporeal membrane oxygenation machine, continuous renal replacement therapies machine, IV pump, tube feeding pump, Foley flow, and cardiopulmonary physiologic monitor. Several nurses made comments about intravenous fluid pumps, "Our patients are on so many medications. An

Table 2
Helpfulness of device/technology alerts/alarms

Device Alarms	Helpful Features	Direct Quotations
Bed exit alarm	Fall notification	That is the one that most people will go running for cuz a patient could have fallen.
Cardiopulmonary physiologic monitor	Abnormal value notification	Even the annoying alarms, I think they [cardiac alarms] are important.... They alert you when somebody's blood pressure is low or high or heart rate is low or high or a rhythm changed.
	Organ function Indication	Keep their [patients'] blood pressure up to a safe level where they're perfusing their brain and their kidneys ... if they're very labile, it'll let me know. ... You can set it [parameter] to a very tight pressure of 65 the whole day, you can make that happen. It's just safety. Withdraw of care - you don't wanna turn the monitor off cuz you need to know when they die.
	Monitoring surrogate	Use that as an auditory que for you to get some things done.
CRRT	Therapeutic notification	It will alarm ... one beep to tell you, your bag is empty. Now you need to change it, instead of a constant alarming.... Okay. Time to change the bag. That's a good alarm for me.
ECMO	Emergency alert	I have a more heightened sense of the alarm that I'm listening for. If my ECMO machine goes off, that's something that's emergent I need to address.
IV pump	Therapeutic notification	If it's [IV pump] beeping, it's not running. I have to go make sure cuz all of our drips are important.
Ventilator	Proper functioning equipment	I pay attention to the ventilator alarms a lot more, because they don't have that many false alarms. Even if the patient's coughing, I still need to know that, cuz that means they're operating properly.
	Unable to adjust the volume	We got the new CRRT machines, and they make a completely different noise than they used to, I can't hear it, and I am like, what is that? What is happening? Cuz, the old ones, you recognized when they were loud, but these are so quiet, and there's no way to increase the volume.

(continued on next page)

Table 2 *(continued)*		
Device Alarms	**Helpful Features**	**Direct Quotations**
	Difficulty with visual alerts	It's got lights that go off, but if you're not directly in front of the thing, you don't see the lights. It's got lots of different lights.
	Screen with complex numbers	It's like 30 numbers on the screen, and everyone just pushes next.
EHR	Unimportant alerts	When you're trying to get something charted, and—it's distracting. All it is is a distraction. It's almost never—I can't think of any that are—I feel important.
	Irrelevant alerts	We used to have the ICU one that was the vaccine, the ICU admission vaccine form, or pop-up, whatever, but we don't vaccinate our patients in the ICU 'cause they're in the ICU.
	Frequency of alerts	Has your patient gone out of the country? Which I'm sure has been addressed at least multiple times with this patient… It'll keep reminding you … Does it have to be so often?
	Excessive complexity/too many steps to complete the task	When you do your IV drips, it's like link here, link here and there's 3 pop-ups just to validate some fluids. That's really frustrating. Everyone skips over it. Skip, skip. I'm not gonna link it. It gives you the option of doing that, but it's just in your way. I know it has a purpose. No one uses that purpose. Then there is no purpose… It's just 20 steps…
IV pump	Unnecessary alarms while trouble-shooting the machine	It [alarm sound] keeps coming up and up and up. Like, Oh my gosh. Stop! I can't think about it! I think that's frustrating. I'm trying to fix it. Now you're alarming even louder while I'm trying to fix the problem. That's frustrating.
	Oversensitivity	There's a teeny little bubble in there and it just alarms, and you won't stop til you get the bubble outta the tubing.
	Silence with short duration	You press pause and silence it, but that silence only lasts for so long. By the time you get back with the next bottle, it's started beeping again.
	Noise	It's a very loud and obnoxious alarm.

(continued on next page)

Table 2 (continued)		
Device Alarms	**Helpful Features**	**Direct Quotations**
Tube feeding	Unnecessary irritating sounds	Certain alarms that are extra irritating that I just—if the sound maybe changed, it wouldn't be as grinding on my nerves. The tube feed thing, it just gets me. I will go from the complete opposite corner of the unit to a whole other—the direct caddy corner opposite to silence the alarm, cuz it is that irritating. Meeeeeeeeeeee forever. It kills me.... It's so awful. I know that it's telling me something important. My tube feed is empty. You need to change the bag. Does it have to be that aggressive?
Multiple devices	Uncoordinated sounds	If they all came out the same speaker or something cuz they all come from so many different places. Sometimes it's hard.
	Sound alike Bathroom and staff assist alarm	Bathroom [assist] alarm and staff assist alarm sounded alike

Abbreviations: CRRT, continuous renal replacement therapies; ECMO, extracorporeal membrane oxygenation; EHR, electronic health record; IV, intravenous.

alarm any time there's a bubble of air or that's running low or if it's occluded in some way. You have literally 12 drips running. You can be alarming all the time." "The constant ding…" and "It won't stop." Other auditory sounds in the ICU environment that critical care nurses identified as auditory alarms included bathroom call light alarms, code blue alarms, nurse call lights, phones, and speakers of alarms in the hallway.

Visual Alerts/Alarms

Participants identified 3 main sources of visual alarms/alerts in the ICU, namely cardio-pulmonary physiologic monitor, EHR, and nurse call light, with most comments surrounding EHR. "It's a little pop-up box that comes up. Usually [they are] like admissions stuff that wasn't done … Those are annoying … I'll go through it again with my patient and everything's good. I check everything off and the message keeps popping up still. Every time you open their chart, it's there…You have to say okay or cancel or Remind me in 4 hours."

Helpfulness of Alerts/Alarms

Participants were further inquired about helpfulness of auditory and visual alarms/ alerts during focus group interviews and their responses were categorized by device in **Table 2**. A statement agreed to by all of the participants was "the ones that you hear a lot of are normally the less helpful ones." Nonetheless, each alarm mentioned was understood as helpful and necessary.

Device/Technology Barriers Contributing to Sensory Overload

Critical care nurses mentioned several device/technology barriers, specifically related to device alarms/alerts, that contribute to sensory overload in the work setting

Table 3
Device/technology barriers specifically related to alerts/alarms

Device	Barriers	Descriptions
Cardiopulmonary physiologic monitor	Unable to silence alarms	In the cardiac world, our patients have very irregular rhythms. All kinds of rhythms all the time. It's very abnormal, but for us, it's almost normal. There's no way to silence the alarm. It's just on all the time, even though we try to turn certain parameters off and can't because of the nature of our patient population.
	Difficult to adjust alarms	If your patient keeps alarming VT because they had 3 PVCs in a row and that patient's having those all the time, in theory, you're supposed to be able to go and change the PVCs, so it doesn't alarm unless you have more than 6 in a row, but we've done that and sometimes that still doesn't work and it'll still alarm for us...there's nothing you can do to change it except ignore.
	Unable to recognize nontextbook rhythms	The problem is the limitations of the monitor and not being able to recognize certain rhythms and a patient's normal. Or even if it's an abnormal rhythm, they're just—it only seems to be able to read certain rhythms, like textbook rhythms... When it's not a textbook rhythm, I think it just recognizes it as a lethal rhythm and there's nothing you can do about it.
	Unable to recognize baseline rhythms	If it could recognize my patient's normal rhythm and be able to differentiate that from an abnormal rhythm. This is my patient's norm, and maybe that is frequent PVCs, a-fib. It doesn't look like a normal rhythm...the monitors actually genuinely only know the textbook rhythms, and there's some patients that are not—that do not fall in that category, but that's their norm, and that's okay, and the monitor will not accept it.
	Too sensitive	Whereas the cardiac alarms, they're always going off. Sometimes I tune those out more.
	Requiring frequent acknowledgment	Every little run of an abnormal rhythm, I have to go and acknowledge it every single time.
	Unable to sense motion artifacts	If you could adjust the sensitivity of some of them because a lotta these machines are designed for people that don't move. If somebody moves much, then the machine will think they're in v-tach [ventricular tachycardia] when they just turned, sneezing or doin' the wiggles.
	Relearn function not effective	I had a patient a little while ago who was having irregular heartbeats every few seconds. I cannot get the machine to relearn the rhythm to know that this is normal, so the entire night, I couldn't get anything done. It was a very busy patient that I was in and out of the room all the time. It would just not stop.

(continued on next page)

Device	Barriers	Descriptions
Table 3 *(continued)*		
	Arrhythmia alarms sound the same	On the arrhythmia alarms, they all sound the same. I don't know if it's just one single PVC or if they're in VTach [ventricular tachycardia] … In cardiovascular ICU, I don't need to know every time a patient throws a PVC, cuz it's gonna happen all the time. Then I get fatigue, so that when they do have a nice run V tach, I don't pay attention to it, cuz they all sound the same.
CRRT	Unable to stop alarms	When the CRRT machine is telling you that your pressure's high, and you're trying to fix it, and it keeps on beeping, and you silence it, and it keeps on—after a while it beeps at you again, that makes me nervous.
	Code blue alarm and bathroom assist alarm	The code (code blue) alarm changed on our unit. The one that sounds like a bathroom alarm. That is so irritating, because if someone goes to the bathroom and pulls the call light for help in the bathroom, it sounds as an emergency… People are running. I actually don't think there is a difference. I think they sound exactly the same.
	CRRT alarm and ECMO alarm	The CRRT machine changed alarms. At first it was awful, because now it sounds exactly like our ECMO machine.

Abbreviations: CRRT, continuous renal replacement therapies; ECMO, extracorporeal membrane oxygenation; EHR, electronic health record; ICU, intensive care unit; IV, intravenous; PVC, premature ventricular contraction.

(**Table 3**). The majority of barriers discussed by participants centered on cardiopulmonary physiologic monitor; as one participant stated, "the cardiac alarms and the tube feeding alarms are the worst." The comments centered on the inability to adjust the alarm or to heighten its specificity, "The problem is the limitations of the monitor and not being able to recognize certain rhythms and a patient's normal…When it's not a textbook rhythm, I think it just recognizes it as a lethal rhythm and there's nothing you can do about it." Another nurse noted in resignation, "If your patient keeps alarming VT [ventricular tachycardia] because they had 3 PVCs [premature ventricular contractions] in a row and that patient's having those all the time, in theory, you're supposed to be able to go and change the PVCs, so it doesn't alarm unless you have more than six in a row, but we've done that and sometimes that still doesn't work and it'll still alarm for us…there's nothing you can do to change it except ignore it."

Of the many devices, the most identified device/technology barriers were surrounding poor user-centered functionalities of cardiopulmonary physiologic monitor. These include being unable to silence alarms, difficulty adjusting alarms, being unable to recognize nontextbook rhythms, being unable to recognize baseline rhythms, being too sensitive, requiring frequent acknowledgment, unable to sense motion artifacts, relearn function not effective, and arrhythmia alarms sound alike.

DISCUSSION

ICUs are unique, complex, and dynamic environments where many technological de-vices assist in the care of critically ill patients with newer devices constantly added. The blinking lights, various alarm noises, and noises from other machines working without a pause all contribute to the hostile working environment of the ICU.[1] Under such difficult working conditions, sensory overload can affect the physical and mental health of critical care nurses and their ability to provide care to critically ill patients. Data from this focus group study provide insights into how auditory and visual alarms/alerts associated with the multitude of medical devices/technologies in the ICU contrib-uted to heightened sensory overload among critical care nurses. Results from this study may inform future research of regarding sensory overload related to medical technology.

There are different types of workload: quantitative (amount of work), qualitative (complexity of the work),[16] cognitive, and physical. Cognitive workload is related to the need for ICU nurses to process information, often very quickly. Physical workload is related particularly to the tasks and their physical characteristics, the availability of devices, and so on. The qualitative workload of critical care nurses is related to the rapid pace of knowledge and implementation of new technologies and devices.[3] Alarms from sophisticated technology add to cognitive, physical, quantitative, and qualitative workloads of critical care nurses.[17] Understanding how medical technolo-gies can contribute to workload is critical for developing interventions aimed at reducing (or managing) workload and its impact on critical care nurses.

Critical care nurses encounter enormous numbers and types of alarms. These alarms come from different devices and are not coordinated. Alarms from cardiopul-monary physiologic monitors, ventilators, and IV pumps were identified by critical care nurses as contributing most to their sensory overload and yet these alarms were also deemed the most helpful ones at work. Of these devices, most identified device/tech-nology barriers were surrounding poor user-centered functionalities (ie, the ability to adjust, reprogram, etc) of cardiopulmonary physiologic monitors. Other research has reported that critical care nurses had attributed their frustration to alarms owing to poor usability of the complex alarm devices, specifically the cardiopulmonary moni-toring systems.[18,19] Even the newer cardiac monitors are viewed by nurses to be "very complex and not user friendly."[18]

Cardiopulmonary physiologic monitors are also known to be overly sensitive with high numbers of clinically irrelevant false alarms. In an observational study, 41% of crisis alarms with highest clinical priority solicited no immediate nursing response.[9] Such reduction in the behavioral or physiologic response to a stimulus that occurs with repeated exposure to that stimulus (an alert) is referred to as habituation, a human factor principle. The phenomenon of habituation has important implications for the design and implementation of alerts/alarms and highlights the necessity to reduce false alarm rates in alerting systems.[20] Even though a pulse oximeter is known to cause false-positive alarms most frequently,[21] alarms from a pulse oximeter were not mentioned to be a contributor to sensory overload by this group of critical care nurses.

Ventilator-associated alarms are often used by critical care nurses as an indicator of proper functioning equipment and no barrier for contributing to sensory overload was identified in this group of ICU nurses. IV pump alarms are deemed helpful for critical care nurses to know the array of IV drips administered are properly running and yet, barriers to IV pump alarms are associated with unnecessary alarms while trouble-shooting the machine, being overly sensitive, a silence function with too short in dura-tion, and loud and obnoxious alarm sounds.

Alerts/alarms from EHR and medication dispensing systems contribute little to sensory overload and are not experienced as helpful. Common barriers specifically related to EHR alerts/alarms included unimportant alerts, irrelevant alerts, high frequency of alerts, and excessive complexity. Excessive complexity is associated with the classic human factors dilemmas of too many steps to complete the task, nonintuitive actions, and/or the actions being too time consuming.[22]

Acoustic Profiles and Integration of Auditory Alarms

To meet operator's needs, sounds must be (1) unique in the surrounding sound environment, (2) easily discriminated from one another, (3) convey the right level of urgency in relation to a degree of priority, and (4) sufficiently audible to be detected but should not be deafening or prevent communication among team members.[23] Critical care nurses identified several alarms in the ICU that make identical or nearly identical sounds regardless of their priority. Sound alike was found in bathroom assist and nurse call lights, bathroom assist call lights and code blue alarms, and alarms from continuous renal replacement therapies and extracorporeal membrane oxygenation machines. Sound alarms are intended to help reduce the nurses' workload during periods of intense activity by attracting nurses' attention. However, it is common to have 30 or so alarms dedicated to monitor a single patient in the ICU and even experienced nurses have difficulty identifying the source of an alarm.[24] Existing alarms embedded in current medical technologies fail to achieve the purpose of reducing nurses' workload. In reality, these alarms are too numerous, too loud or irritating, do not convey the right degree of urgency, and lack systematic integration because each sound alarm is designed in isolation.

In an ICU environment where patient status is constantly changing, multitasking is normal, and the use of multiple medical technologies is inevitable. Interface with complex medical technologies and noise pollution from these alarm-generating devices in the ICU are significant predictors of burnout in critical care nurses. Alarm systems embedded in existing medical devices are far from intuitive and user friendly, so that these necessary alarm mechanisms became sources of sensory overload among critical care nurses. Findings from this study demonstrated that user-centered and integrated improvements in alarm systems associated with an array of medical devices in the ICU is much needed. Such effort has great potential to lead to an improved physical work environment by decreasing noise pollution, decrease technology-related stress and burnout among critical care nurses, and ultimately, improve patient care and safety.

ACKNOWLEDGMENTS

The authors would like to thank Usha Menon, PhD, RN, FAAN, who served as the focus group facilitator for this study.

REFERENCES

1. Donchin Y, Seagull FJ. The hostile environment of the intensive care unit. Curr Opin Crit Care 2002;8(4):316–20.
2. Foglia DC, Grassley JS, Zeigler VL. Factors that influence pediatric intensive care unit nurses to leave their jobs. Crit Care Nurs Q 2010;33(4):302–16.
3. Schaufeli WB, Keijsers GJ, Reis Miranda D. Burnout, technology use, and ICU-performance. Organizational risk factors for job stress 1995;12:259–71.
4. Crickmore R. A review of stress in the intensive care unit. Intensive Care Nurs 1987;3(1):19–27.

5. Poncet MC, Toullic P, Papazian L, et al. Burnout syndrome in critical care nursing staff. Am J Respir Crit Care Med 2007;175(7):698–704.
6. O'Brien-Pallas L, Murphy GT, Shamian J, et al. Impact and determinants of nurse turnover: a pan-Canadian study. J Nurs Manag 2010;18(8):1073–86.
7. Sawatzky JA. Stress in critical care nurses: actual and perceived. Heart Lung 1996;25(5):409–17.
8. Grumet GW. Pandemonium in the modern hospital. N Engl J Med 1993;328(6): 433–7.
9. Varpio L, Kuziemsky C, MacDonald C, et al. The helpful or hindering effects of in-hospital patient monitor alarms on nurses: a qualitative analysis. Comput Inform Nurs 2012;30(4):210–7.
10. Epp K. Burnout in critical care nurses: a literature review. Dynamics 2012;23(4): 25–31.
11. Topf M, Dillon E. Noise-induced stress as a predictor of burnout in critical care nurses. Heart Lung 1988;17(5):567–74.
12. Jones DM, Davies D. Individual and group differences in the response to noise. In: Noise and society. Chichester (UK): Wiley; 1984. p. 125–53.
13. Broadbent D. Differences and interactions between stresses. Q J Exp Psychol 1963;15(3):205–11.
14. Loeb M. Noise and human efficiency. John Wiley & Sons; 1986.
15. Canadian Nurses Association. Nurse fatigue and patient safety. Ottawa (Ontario): Canadian Nurses Association; 2010.
16. Frankenhaeuser M, Gardell B. Underload and overload in working life: outline of a multidisciplinary approach. J Human Stress 1976;2(3):35–46.
17. Carayon P, Alvarado CJ, Systems Engineering Initiative for Patient Safety. Workload and patient safety among critical care nurses. Crit Care Nurs Clin North Am 2007;19(2):121–9.
18. Sowan AK, Tarriela AF, Gomez TM, et al. Nurses' perceptions and practices toward clinical alarms in a transplant cardiac intensive care unit: exploring key issues leading to alarm fatigue. JMIR Hum Factors 2015;2(1):e3.
19. Drews F. Patient monitors in critical care: lessons for improvement. In: Henriksen K, BJ, Keyes MA, et al, editors. Advances in patient safety: new directions and alternative approaches, vol. 3: performance and tools. Rockville (MD): Agency for Healthcare Research and Quality (US); 2008.
20. Phansalkar S, Edworthy J, Hellier E, et al. A review of human factors principles for the design and implementation of medication safety alerts in clinical information systems. J Am Med Inform Assoc 2010;17(5):493–501.
21. Tsien CL, Fackler JC. Poor prognosis for existing monitors in the intensive care unit. Crit Care Med 1997;25(4):614–9.
22. Henriksen K, Battles JB, Keyes MA, et al. Fault tree analysis of clinical alarms. J Clin Eng 2008;85–94.
23. Guillaume A. Intelligent auditory alarms. In: Hermann T, Hunt A, Neuhoff JG, editors. The sonification handbook. Berlin: Logos Publishing House; 2011. p. 493–508.
24. Cropp AJ, Woods LA, Raney D, et al. Name that tone. The proliferation of alarms in the intensive care unit. Chest 1994;105(4):1217–20.

Critical Care Nurses' Cognitive Ergonomics Related to Medical Device Alarms

Shu-Fen Wung, PhD, RN, ACNP-BC[a],*,
Marilyn Rose Schatz, DNP, RN, ACNP-BC[b]

KEYWORDS

- Decision making • Monitor alarms • Alarm fatigue • Intensive care • Human factors

KEY POINTS

- Intensive care nurses integrate multiple factors into consideration when deciding how quickly or even whether an alarm will be responded to.
- Difficulties encountered in responding to alarms included low staffing, multiple job responsibilities, and competing priority tasks.
- Less experienced nurses tend to rely on monitor alarms to alert them to a patient problem.
- Less experienced nurses are more tolerant of alarms sounding owing to a lower threshold of comfort with resetting or silencing alarms.
- Future studies should include effective use of alarm-related equipment trainings and/or innovative user-centered alarm management clinical decision support systems to enhance intuitive nurse–device interactions.

INTRODUCTION

Acute care nurses are responsible for the safety of critically ill patients around the clock in the increasingly complex technology-rich intensive care units (ICUs) by making distinctions between clinical changes that warrant emergent intervention and those that do not.[1] In this high-pressure work environment, numerous devices, often complicated, are commonly used to enable continuous measurements of the physiologic function of the patient and function of the medical devices.[2] To increase safety, alarms are embedded in almost every device in the ICU to alert critical care nurses of potential problems early so they can institute appropriate interventions. Nurses are

Disclosure Statement: There is no commercial or financial conflicts of interest for all authors. There is no grant or other financial support used for the study.

[a] Biobehavioral Health Science Division, The University of Arizona College of Nursing, 1305 North Martin Avenue, Tucson, AZ 85721- 0203, USA; [b] Pulmonary Consultants of Mesa, 6750 E Baywood Avenue Ste 401, Mesa, AZ 85206, USA
* Corresponding author.
E-mail address: wung@arizona.edu

expected to monitor and respond appropriately to the plethora of pathophysiologic data and alarms produced by the patient and devices.

Ironically, the very alarm systems created to enhance patient safety have become an urgent patient safety concern.[2] Just a bedside cardiopulmonary monitor alone generates 187 audible alarms per bed per day, averaging 1 alarm every 7.7 minutes.[3] To exacerbate the alarm problem further, up to 90% of alarms are deemed false or nonactionable with very few indicating serious clinical events.[4–10] The constant demand to respond to alarms and mistrust of the alarm system owing to high numbers of clinically irrelevant alarms reduce the alertness of the clinicians. Clinicians become accustomed to ignoring false alarms and, as a result, may overlook an alarm that signals a true emergency, producing a phenomenon known as alarm fatigue. Patient injury and death resulting from inadequate attention to alarms have been reported.[11] In addition, silencing alarms is the second most common task performed by nurses, accounting for approximately 16% of a nurse's bedside tasks.[12]

As more tasks are handled by technology, humans are becoming responsible for tasks that require inference, diagnoses, judgment, and decision making.[13] In the ICU, ever-growing and complex technology places nurses at a greater cognitive demand. As defined by the International Ergonomics Association, cognitive ergonomics (or human factors) is "concerned with mental processes, such as perception, memory, reasoning, and motor response, as they affect interactions among humans and other elements of a system. (Relevant topics include mental workload, decision-making, skilled performance, human-computer interaction, human reliability, work stress and training as these may relate to human-system design.)"[14] Decision making, a process that humans use to determine a forward path of action,[15] is 1 of 10 key human factors topics relevant for patient safety.[16] To design an effective alarm management program, we propose to focus on cognitive ergonomics by understanding critical care nurses' cognitive processes, specifically intricacy of decision-making capabilities, related to prioritizing, responding to, and managing medical device alarms in ICU, when under conditions of high uncertainty, time pressure, and risk.

THEORETIC FRAMEWORK

The situated clinical decision-making framework provides a structured approach to analyze nurses' decision making in clinical practice and to guide the selection of relevant strategies to support development of clinical decision making.[17] In this framework, 4 phases have been identified to comprise the clinical decision-making process—cues, judgments, decisions, and evaluation of outcomes.[18] A nurse's clinical decision-making process is triggered by recognition of a cue from the patient, either a response or lack of something expected. Once the initial cue is noticed, the nurse collects additional cues to build an understanding of the situation. Cues can be collected from multiple sources, including patient observation and assessment, statements from patients or others, objective data, and the nurse's intuition. Ongoing cue collection is informed by a nurse's evolving understanding of the situation. For example, when a device alarm sounds, the nurse is cued to a possible change in patient condition. This alarm may trigger a reminder of a comment made by the patient, such as a previous complaint of discomfort. Judgment is defined as the best conclusion that can be reached at a point in time, given the available information. This definition reflects the dynamic process between possible judgements and collected cues. Ongoing cues further informs one's judgment. *Decision* is committing to a course of action, whether it is "waiting and watching" and/or "trying something."[18] The nurse may choose to proceed with a tentative course of action and remain open to revise the actions as new information becomes available. *Evaluation of outcomes* is a reflection on the effectiveness of cue collection, judgment, and decision, and whether further action is indicated. Reflecting on the outcome is an opportunity for clinical improvement and nurses often unconsciously go over their decisions to ensure that the best decision has been made for the patient in that particular situation.[17]

METHODS
Design, Setting, and Sample

This descriptive study aimed at understanding the complexities of the decision-making process related medical device alarms among ICU nurses. A semistructured interview was designed and conducted with a sample of 16 registered nurses from a 30-bed combined medical-surgical, cardiac, and cardiovascular surgical ICU in a 178-bed community hospital. The nurses typically work 12-hour shifts. Eight nurses, 7 women and 1 man, were interviewed from each shift to obtain equal representation from each timeframe.

Because nurses' decision making often evolves with experience,[17] we analyzed decision-making process related to medical device alarm by nurses' clinical experience, advanced beginners and experts. Benner[19] defined an advanced beginner nurse as a person who has experienced actual clinical situations to identify their significant elements and the expert nurse has an instinctive grasp of the situation and can pinpoint the problem without having to consider options that are not useful in a given situation. In this study, advanced beginner and expert were arbitrary defined as having 5 or fewer years and more than 5 years of ICU experience, respectively.

Instrument

Semistructured open-ended interview questions were developed based on decision-making process of the situated clinical decision-making framework and formulated to probe a situation related to device alarm to bring out the cognitive processes used in making a decision. Questions focused on device alarm identification, alarm management, and parameter settings on the monitor. There were total of 15 questions, including cues initiating the decision-making process, judgment on how nurses processed the cues, decisions made after judging the cues, and reflection on areas amenable for improvement, such as training on the monitors or refresher courses on cardiac rhythm interpretation. The content validity of this semistructured interview was supported by 3 doctorally prepared nurse researchers and 3 board-certified acute care nurse practitioners.

Data Collection Protocol

Upon approval from institutions' human subjects protection programs and permission from the study ICU, the purpose of this study was presented at a unit meeting and interested participants were encouraged to contact the researcher. Informed consent was obtained from each nurse before the interview. Each interview was recorded and later transcribed verbatim to ensure completeness of the data.

Data analysis

A content analysis was performed and began with reading and rereading the transcription several times to obtain an overview of the data. General categorization was based on the 4 phases of the clinical decision-making process: cues, judgments, decisions, and evaluation of outcomes. A further analysis of transcript was performed to identify concepts within each of the 4 themes and interpret the meaning of responses to better understand the decision-making process as it related to monitor alarms. Descriptive statistics were used to describe demographic data.

RESULTS
Sample Characteristics

Sixteen ICU nurses participated in the interview. Of these, 38% and 62% were advanced beginners and experts, respectively. The mean age of ICU nurses was 38 ± 11 years (range, 27–60 years), and the mean years of ICU experience was 9 ± 7 years (range, 1.5–21.0 years). Educational preparation of these nurses included 2 with diploma degrees, 5 with an associate degree of nursing, 8 with a bachelor of science in nursing, and 1 with a master's of science in nursing.

Nurses' cognitive ergonomics, specifically decision making related to medical device alarms, are presented herein, according the 4 areas of mental processing (cues, judgments, decisions and evaluation of outcomes) of the situated clinical decision-making framework.

Cues

Alarms in the intensive care unit

Nurses indicated that they felt overwhelmed by monitor alarms, yet, the number of hourly alarms they heard or dealt with varied greatly within the same ICU; only 38% heard more than 5 alarms per hour in their last shift. Of the nurses who heard more than 5 alarms per hour, 80% were expert nurses. An advanced beginner nurse with 1.5 years of ICU experience stated that, "There is always something, whether it is a ventilator or the actual ICU monitors, like the vital sign machine, the SCD [sequential compression device] machine, or the beds. There are always alarms going off every minute or so."

Cues affect timeliness of alarm response

Disregarding years of ICU experience, among nurses interviewed, there was a unified initial response to an alarm: "It needs attention." ICU nurses took multiple factors into consideration when deciding how quickly to respond to alarms. These included the tone of the alarm, priority of other competing activities, and patient status. Factors that determine how fast or even whether an alarm will be responded to often depends more on the volume of the alarm bell than the urgency of the underlying condition. Thirty-three percent of advanced beginner nurses stated that they might ignore the alarm when they are engaged in a higher priority task. "If I am in the middle of an emergent situation, I probably shut a lot of them [alarms] out"; "If I happen to be doing something really really important, I'll let it [alarm] slide." Similarly, expert nurses stated that their timeliness of response to an alarm was determined by the tone of the alarm as well as the patient status. "Well I think all alarms are important, so the high level alerts you always want to check immediately, but I like to get to my alarms as soon as possible." "Any sound you have to do it quickly, because it is alarming for a reason."

Judgment

Judgment on alarm urgency

Nurses interviewed judged the urgency of an alarm based on the tones of the alarm and knowledge of the patient's condition, as well as immediate visualization of the patient. The urgency of an alarm is judged "by the tones of the alarm and my knowledge of the patient's condition," an advanced beginner responded. An expert nurse stated, "Is it a low level alarm? Are my alarm parameters correct? If you have a patient who has been in sinus rhythm [and the heart rates are] in the 80s, and all of a sudden they're in atrial fib [fibrillation] with a [heart] rate of 120, well that needs some pretty direct attention."

Judgment on alarm validity
Nurses gathered information through both visual and auditory means to decide if an alarm is authentic. An advanced beginner stated, "If it's a real alarm, as opposed to artifact, I'd like to look at the patient to see if there are any safety concerns." Responses from experts regarding ways to authenticate an alarm included: "It depends on the alarm. If you look up and see your EKG [electrocardiographic] monitor, does it look like a Vtach [ventricular tachycardia] or Vfib [ventricular fibrillation]? If the patient has an art [arterial] line, do I have a pressure? I correlate those two. If it [EKG monitor] says Vtach and you have a good arterial pressure, then it is probably not Vtach."

Decision

Initial response to an alarm
Both expert and advanced beginner nurses felt they needed to observe the patient as well as assess the alarm validity to accurately make a decision as to whether the alarm warranted interventions. Advanced beginner nurses responded, "To figure out what alarm it is, or where it is coming from [cardiac monitor or other equipment]." "I assess the patient, look at what is alarming, and see if I have enough information after I assess the patient." Responses from expert nurses including, "First I have to look at the alarm to see what it is, but you also have to look at the patient, that is, the important thing"; "Look at the patient, look and see what the alarm is and correlate the two"; and "If it's life threatening, even if it is not your patient, get up and go in there, and see what is going on."

Resetting default alarm parameters
The decision to reset alarm parameters was based on providers' treatment orders, after observing the patient's baseline vital signs, with a change in patient's clinical condition, and the nurses' comfort level. Resetting alarm parameters was done when nurses came on shift once they have assessed their patients. Eighty-six percent of nurses interviewed stated that they understood the need to set parameters specifically to their patients' baseline and 50% of expert nurses would observe the patient before adjusting the parameters. Responses from advanced beginners included: "It always depends on the patient. I try to figure out [the parameters] based on if the patient is asymptomatic and if this [parameters] is normal for the patient." "If the patient became unstable, like if the patient coded, you would just start from scratch because they are no longer at their baseline." Responses from expert nurses related to resetting monitor parameters included: "The only time I would do that [resetting the default alarm parameters] is once I know their [the patient's] baseline." "After watching the monitor for a couple of hours and seeing which alarms are going off more often and where my patient's normality is." "It depends on what is ok with the physician. If the physician is ok with the patient's [heart rate] running in the 130s... Maybe he [the patient] just needs more fluids. Maybe I'd up them [the parameters] until they [patient's vital signs] came back to normal." "When they [the parameters] are not appropriate for that particular patient, I'd like to customize monitor alarms based on my patient's [unique condition]." One expert nurse interviewed did not see the need to adjust monitor parameters and another indicated that nurses were not allowed to adjust alarms unless given specific parameters from the physician. "Reset the parameters? I don't think we reset them, do we? I don't reset them." When inquiring about parameter settings that made the nurse uncomfortable, an advanced beginner responded: "It depends on the situation. I am actually pretty anxious. If it is normal for the patient or

physician has specified otherwise, then it's okay to go out of the [default] parameters. if there is too big of a deviation [from patient's normal or default parameters], I will get a second and third opinion." An expert nurse responded: "Settings that would not allow me to intervene in a timely manner: a pressure that is too low, respiratory rates that are too low."

Frequent false alarms related to blood pressure
All nurses felt blood pressure readings needed to be accurate and would intervene to minimize false alarms often by troubleshooting the equipment or blood pressure acquisition site. An advanced beginner responded: "Well, you need to figure out why it [BP] is not true. If the A-line [arterial-line] is not patent, then you try to adjust it, fix it or pull it. You just can't have inaccurate values recorded in the medical record." An expert nurse responded: "I would try to troubleshoot the problem to see why I am getting the false alarms and reset my parameters on my monitor."

Frequent false alarms related to heart rate or arrhythmia
For frequent false heart rate or arrhythmia alarms, nurses would determine if there is a problem with the monitoring system, a restless patient, or the parameters not set appropriately for that patient. Thirteen percent of nurses indicated that they do not attend to these alarms, allow them to sound, or silence them. A nurse with 2.5 years of ICU experience stated, "Look at the patient, are they moving around? Check the placement of the leads and go from there." A nurse with 5 years of ICU experience stated, "I wouldn't do anything, continue to monitor them [the alarms]." Responses from expert nurses included: "You can silence [the alarm], like if the patient is in A fib [atrial fibrillation]. You can turn off the yellow alarms, the irregular rate one." "Are the parameters right? Are the electrodes right? Are they [electrodes] in the right position?"

Frequent false alarms related to pulse oximetry
Nurses indicated that false pulse oximetry readings are frequent problems. Solutions included changing the probe sensor to a site with good perfusion, improve perfusion by warming the extremity, or changing the probe sensor, cable, or monitor module. An advanced beginner nurse responded, "I would try to keep moving it [oximetry probe sensor] on the patient until it [pulse oximetry] wasn't alarming and was reading what seems to be correct." Expert nurses also considered patient treatments that could interfere with pulse oximetry reading, such as vasopressor use. An expert nurse replied, "Pulse oximetry is kind of a nightmare in and of itself. you know- Is it a good sensor? Is it in the right place? Is it on the non-dominant arm? is it an old cuff? Are they [patients] on pressors [vasopressors]?

Decision on disabling alarms
The level of an alarm (eg, crisis, advisory), presence of a backup warning mechanism, patients' clinical status, and the nurses' comfort level are factors taken into account while judging if an alarm may be disabled. For example, 62% of expert nurses would disable the apnea alarm on the cardiac monitor in a ventilated patient and use the ventilator apnea alarm as a backup. However, 25% of nurses stated that they would never disable an alarm unless the patient was transitioning to step-down or comfort care. All nurses interviewed expressed that disabling alarms on patients who are placed on comfort care is an acceptable practice, although 60% of advanced beginner nurses were hesitant about disabling any alarm. All nurses indicated that alarms for blood pressure, arterial line, and oxygen saturation should not be disabled at any time. An advanced beginner responded, "No, [I do not disable alarms] even

when they keep going off … I am scared if the one time I disabled it [the alarm] something really bad is going to happen and I don't want that." Expert nurses' responses related to disabling monitor alarms included: "I do, yes I do. I disable respiration alarms [on the cardiac monitor] if they [patients] are on the ventilator because there is no point to even having those [alarms]." "The only exception [I disabled the alarm] was a patient placed on comfort care because the alarms were irritating to the family and did not require intervention."

Decision on seeking consultation
Regardless of the duration of ICU experience, all nurses interviewed expressed that they do not hesitate to consult a colleague when the patient's safety is in question. When nurses are unsure if an alarm is real, they tended to err on the side of caution, perform additional assessments, and obtain a second opinion. Advanced beginner nurses were more likely to call for help from another nurse or the charge nurse. Expert nurses tended to take more time to assess the situation before calling for help. Responses from advanced beginner nurses included, "When I need help, if the patient is getting sicker real fast and I cannot manage the patient alone," "If I am unsure of a certain course of action or if I come across something new, I try to get their [colleagues'] inputs. There are a lot of experienced nurses around here. I go to them." An expert nurse stated, "When I question my own ability to figure out what is going on, or if what I thought was going on was true but I did not know what to do about it." In addition, nurses' trust in a colleague's judgment is reliant on their previous experience with that person in a critical situation. They often solicited guidance from someone with whom they have had a positive working experience. "You learn who to trust by working with them and know their level of expertise. You also learn who not to trust."

Evaluation

Barriers to response to alarms
Difficulties encountered in responding to alarms included low staffing, multiple job responsibilities, and competing priority tasks. Responses from advanced beginner nurses included: "Sometimes it is just impossible to manage alarms because we are low staffed. I can't even emphasize my frustration with that." "Call lights, multiple alarms going off at one time, and putting orders in. If you are putting in orders on a patient, you block everything out so you can focus." An expert nurse replied, "I have multiple jobs at one time. It is hard for me to physically go to two different areas to respond [to alarms]. When I am in charge, it is not only the alarms in the ICU I have to respond to but also to codes in the whole hospital. Plus, I am in the count. There is only a certain amount of alarms I can respond to."

Consequences of disabling alarms
All nurses interviewed were aware that disabling alarms in ICU patients can have dire consequences. An advanced beginner stated: "I am sure bad things have happened many times before. That is why disabling something [alarms] should not be done lightly… That's why continuity of care is important. Once you know a patient, you are a little more comfortable which alarms you can turn off and which you can't." An expert nurse responded, "Oh yea, absolutely. If you disable them [alarms] you are missing the whole point of an alarm. You can compromise patient safety if you disarm the alarm."

Determination of adequate alarm management
Nurses felt that adequate alarm management can be determined if the alarms sounded are valid, the number of false alarms are decreased, patients are safe, and

patients do not complain about the constant noise and sleep interruption. An advanced beginner nurse responded, "I really judge it [adequacy of alarm management] off how safe I feel the patient is, and how well I feel they are doing. I feel like if the alarms keep going off, something is not right. I have to figure it out." Responses from expert nurses included, "I have had patients tell me that they have gotten more sleep than they have in a while. They actually have not gotten sleep because of what is going on with their alarms," "Do I have many false alarms? Can I believe the ones that I have? ... Because for me I should always believe my alarms until proven otherwise."

Training received on monitors
Only 25% of nurses (n = 4) stated that they were familiar with monitors used in the study ICU and among these, only 50% (n = 2) had formal training. All nurses stated that they were shown the "basics" by their preceptors during orientation and this brief training was limited to the expertise and experience of their preceptors. "I didn't get any training on how to use the monitors. During my orientation it was - these are the monitors, here is where you silence them, that was about it." "When we first opened [this hospital], they trained us on [how to use] the monitors." "I had used these monitors a long time ago but basically you only get what your preceptor taught you." Several nurses also expressed that lack of formal training with monitors was also an issue in their prior employment.

DISCUSSION

Decision making is "the process of reaching a judgment or choosing an option, sometimes called a course of action, to meet the needs of a given situation."[20] Across different occupations, examples of the importance of decision-making skills for safe task performance are abundant[20]; however, research on decision making in health care during task execution, especially under high pressure and uncertain conditions, is needed. Herein we have investigated individual nurse's cognition, specifically regarding decision making related to device alarms, in real-world contexts.

The proliferation of sophisticated physiologic monitoring and treatment devices has become an integral part of intensive care. Nurses indicated that they felt overwhelmed by device alarms and these alarms are also disruptive to patients. Yet, the number of hourly alarms they heard or dealt with varied greatly within the same ICU, with only 38% heard more than 5 alarms per hour in their last shift. Pervasive low urgency and false alarms can become ongoing background noise to the point that the staff is not fully aware of the sound.[21] If the nurse experienced a history of false alarms with a particular device, the alarm may be ignored easily if it went off inappropriately.[21] Funk and colleagues[22] infer that excessive alarm racket can become "white noise" that nurses ignore or rely on the monitor technician to inform them of important alarms. The low numbers of monitor alarms heard by some nurses in the present study may be owing to nurses tuning out white noise and only hearing alarms with high urgency or rely on the monitor technician to inform them of important alarms. A nurse with 20 years of ICU experience reasoned, "The fact that we have a monitor technician now in the ICU I think most people really don't pay any attention [to the alarms], including myself unless it [the alarm] is specifically from my patient."

ICU nurses integrate multiple factors into considerations when deciding how quickly or even whether an alarm will be responded to. These included the tone, duration, and type of the alarm, the priority of other competing activities, adequacy of staffing, knowledge of patient acuity, and years of ICU experience. Nurses do not judge the urgency of an alarm in isolation. They integrate their knowledge of the patient's condition and immediate visualization of the patient into their judgment. The nurses felt that the ability to make such judgment is enhanced by knowledge of the monitoring system and situational experience.

Tone, Duration, and Type of Alarm

Audible alarms can improve patient safety when they are used properly in the work environment. Factors that affect nurses' promptness to respond to the alarm often depends on the volume, duration and type of the alarm sound. Thirteen percent of nurses indicated that they do not attend to heart rate and arrhythmia alarms, allow them to sound, or silence them, likely owing to the high frequency of false alarms.

Audible alarms, like the ones embedded in the medical devices, are considered abstract alarms. The connection of these abstract alarms with urgency is learned when the operator (nurse) knows what the alarm means and reacts accordingly.[23] Cropp and colleagues[24] tested whether ICU staff could quickly recognize life-threatening alarms better than the less urgent ones, by sound alone, and reported that critical alarms were correctly identified only one-half the time and noncritical sounds only 40% of the time by ICU personnel. Nurses with more than 1 year of experience in the ICU could recognize better the noncritical sounds, but not the critical ones. Cropp and colleagues[24] concluded that the myriad of alarms regularly occurring in the ICU are too much for even experienced ICU staff to quickly discern. Trainings to include a full range of alerting sounds that ICU nurses are expected to encounter would be beneficial in the ICU setting.

Competing Activities and Staffing Issues

Low staffing, multiple job responsibilities, and competing priority tasks are barriers for ICU nurses to respond to alarms. When the nurse is genuinely too busy with tasks of equal or greater importance, it is not surprising that they are unable to respond to the new alarm. In the present study, one-third of advanced beginner nurses indicated that they might ignore the alarm when they are engaged in a higher priority task. This prioritization could be the result of generally inadequate staffing or an excess of simultaneous or near simultaneous events.[21] When workload gets high and there are too many competing demands, adequate staffing and workload evaluation should be a part of effective alarm management strategies.

Intensive Care Unit Experience

All nurses felt that they need to validate the alarm by correlating their visualization of the patient and the types of alarms. When nurses are unsure if an alarm is real, they tended to err on the side of caution. ICU nurses with less experience tend to appropriately consult a colleague sooner, whereas nurses with more experience tend to perform additional assessment before calling for help. The first priority on the management of false alarms was to ensure the patient is safe before trouble shooting the equipment, including changing electrocardiographic electrodes and pulse oximeter probes or probe sites.

Less experienced nurses tend to rely on monitor alarms to alert them to a patient problem and are more tolerant of alarms sounding owing to a lower threshold of comfort with resetting or silencing alarms. Their hesitancy to disable any alarm is likely due to a lack of exposure to repeat patterns that enhance their judgment capability.[25] Novice nurses' decision making characteristically tends toward rule-based thinking, with a focus on task completion or responding to discrete patient issues, and thus they are more likely to ignore an alarm if they are engaged in a task that is deemed higher in priority.

Expert nurses tend to integrate patterns and factual informational cues with situational experience to inform their decisions[25] and are more likely to view patient situations as a whole and within context.[26] It has also been reported that expert nurses make a judgment more quickly in a critical clinical situation without having to waste time considering options that are not helpful.[25] In this case, nurses with extensive ICU experience tend to correlate tone and duration of alarm with knowledge of patient condition to guide their response to an alarm and consider extensive clinical variables when troubleshooting false alarms (eg, vasopressor diminishing perfusion, which interferes with pulse oximetry readings). In addition, expert nurses are more comfortable than novice nurses to reset alarm parameters, and such a practice is often done after nurses have the chance to assess their patients and their individualized baselines after assumed care.

Inadequate training on alarm devices

Data from the present study revealed a very concerning practice issue: the majority of ICU nurses indicated that they were unfamiliar with the cardiac monitors used and had little or no formal training with the cardiac monitors. The brief training received by critical care nurses was limited to the expertise and experience of their preceptors, a common theme emerged as "these are the monitors, here is where you silence them...." This finding is consistent with prior report in that critical care nurses attribute their frustration to alarms owing to poor usability of the complex alarm devices, specifically the cardiopulmonary monitoring systems.[27,28] Nurses reported that newer cardiac monitors to be "very complex and not user friendly" and it takes a long time for one to feel comfortable interacting with physiologic monitors.[27]

"Inadequate staff training on the proper use and functioning of (alarm-related) equipment" has been recognized by the Joint Commission.[29] Nurses interviewed in the present study felt a formal training would strengthen their ability to manage alarms. However, traditional group-based, one-time training on complex alarm-equipped monitoring devices has been reported to be inadequate to decrease alarm burden.[30] Future studies on alarm management should focus on effective use of alarm-related equipment trainings and/or innovative user-centered alarm management clinical decision support systems to enhance intuitive nurse–device interactions.

Study Limitations

A limitation of this study is the small sample of nurses from a single ICU. Participants from multiple ICUs would enrich the findings. In addition, Benner's definition of advanced beginner was a nurse who has had prior experience in actual clinical situations, whereas the competent nurse has had 2 to 3 years of experience in the same job situation and is able to demonstrate ability and confidence in their decisions.[19] Owing to the small sample size, advanced beginners and competent nurses were combined as "advanced beginners." Although some differences have emerged in phases of clinical decision-making process related to alarm management between advanced beginners and expert nurses, it is likely that arbitrary years of clinical experience may not fully reflect competency.

SUMMARY

Noise pollution caused by excessive monitor alarms and the hazards of alarm fatigue is well-known. This study uniquely gained insight into the intricacy of the ICU nurses' critical decision process when responding to device alarms using the situated clinical decision-making framework, namely, constructs of cues, judgment, decision, and evaluation, with a semistructured interview. We found that ICU nurses integrate multiple subjective and objective factors to decide their responses to monitor alarms and their management. Nurses with fewer years of experience are more tolerant of alarms sounding owing to a lower threshold of comfort with resetting or silencing alarms, whereas ICU nurses with more extensive experience are more comfortable resetting alarm limits to the patient's baseline. Understanding the decision-making process used by nurses can guide the development of policies and learning experiences that are crucial clinical support for alarm management. Optimizing nursing orientation to include structured training with monitors can improve alarm management, decrease the number of false alarms, decrease alarm fatigue, and ultimately improve patient safety and patient outcomes.

REFERENCES

1. Ebright PR, Patterson ES, Chalko BA, et al. Understanding the complexity of registered nurse work in acute care settings. J Nurs Adm 2003;33(12):630–8.
2. Donchin Y, Seagull FJ. The hostile environment of the intensive care unit. Curr Opin Crit Care 2002;8(4):316–20.
3. Drew BJ, Harris P, Zegre-Hemsey JK, et al. Insights into the problem of alarm fatigue with physiologic monitor devices: a comprehensive observational study of consecutive intensive care unit patients. PLoS One 2014;9(10):e110274.
4. Atzema C, Schull MJ, Borgundvaag B, et al. ALARMED: adverse events in low-risk patients with chest pain receiving continuous electrocardiographic monitoring in the emergency department. A pilot study. Am J Emerg Med 2006; 24(1):62–7.
5. Lawless ST. Crying wolf: false alarms in a pediatric intensive care unit. Crit Care Med 1994;22(6):981–5.
6. Tsien CL, Fackler JC. Poor prognosis for existing monitors in the intensive care unit. Crit Care Med 1997;25(4):614–9.
7. Chambrin MC, Ravaux P, Calvelo-Aros D, et al. Multicentric study of monitoring alarms in the adult intensive care unit (ICU): a descriptive analysis. Intensive Care Med 1999;25(12):1360–6.
8. Imhoff M, Kuhls S, Gather U, et al. Smart alarms from medical devices in the OR and ICU. Best Pract Res Clin Anaesthesiol 2009;23(1):39–50.
9. O'Carroll TM. Survey of alarms in an intensive therapy unit. Anaesthesia 1986; 41(7):742–4.
10. Talley LB, Hooper J, Jacobs B, et al. Cardiopulmonary monitors and clinically significant events in critically ill children. Biomed Instrum Technol 2011;(Suppl): 38–45.
11. Weil KM. Alarming monitor problems. Nursing 2009;39(9):58.
12. Gorges M, Markewitz BA, Westenskow DR. Improving alarm performance in the medical intensive care unit using delays and clinical context. Anesth Analg 2009; 108(5):1546–52.
13. Militello LG, Hutton RJ. Applied cognitive task analysis (ACTA): a practitioner's toolkit for understanding cognitive task demands. Ergonomics 1998;41(11): 1618–41.
14. International Ergonomics Association. Available at: http://www.iea.cc/whats/index.html. Accessed December 8, 2017.
15. Hassall M, Xiao T. Human factors and ergonomics. 2015.
16. Flin R, Winter J, Cakil Sarac MR. Human factors in patient safety: review of topics and tools. World Health Organization; 2009. p. 2.

17. Gillespie M. Using the situated clinical decision-making framework to guide analysis of nurses' clinical decision-making. Nurse Educ Pract 2010;10(6):333–40.
18. Gillespie M, Peterson BL. Helping novice nurses make effective clinical decisions: the situated clinical decision-making framework. Nurs Educ Perspect 2009;30(3):164–70.
19. Benner P. From novice to expert. Am J Nurs 1982;82(3):402–7.
20. Flin RH, O'Connor P, Crichton M. Safety at the sharp end: a guide to non-technical skills. Boca Raton (FL): CRC Press; 2008.
21. Hyman WA, Johnson E. Fault tree analysis of clinical alarms. J Clin Eng 2008;85–94.
22. Funk M, Clark JT, Bauld TJ, et al. Attitudes and practices related to clinical alarms. American journal of critical care : an official publication. Aliso Viejo (CA): American Association of Critical-Care Nurses; 2014;23(3):e9–18.
23. Guillaume A. Intelligent auditory alarms. In: Hermann T, Hunt A, Neuhoff JG, editors. The sonification handbook. Berlin: Logos Publishing House; 2011. p. 493–508.
24. Cropp AJ, Woods LA, Raney D, et al. Name that tone. The proliferation of alarms in the intensive care unit. Chest 1994;105(4):1217–20.
25. Crandall B, Klein G, Hoffman R. Working minds: a practitioner's guide to cognitive task analysis. Cambridge (MA): The MIT Press; 2006.
26. Benner PE, Tanner CA, Chesla CA. Expertise in nursing practice: caring, clinical judgment, and ethics. New York: Springer Publishing Company; 1996.
27. Sowan AK, Tarriela AF, Gomez TM, et al. Nurses' perceptions and practices toward clinical alarms in a transplant cardiac intensive care unit: exploring key issues leading to alarm fatigue. JMIR Hum Factors 2015;2(1):e3.
28. Drews F. Patient monitors in critical care: lessons for improvement. In: Henriksen K, Battles JB, Keyes MA, et al, editors. Advances in patient safety: new directions and alternative approaches: performance and tools, vol. 3. Rockville (MD): Agency for Healthcare Research and Quality (US); 2008. p. 1–13.
29. Alert SE. New alert promotes medical device alarm safety in hospitals. Joint Commission Perspectives 2013.
30. Sowan AK, Gomez TM, Tarriela AF, et al. Changes in default alarm settings and standard in-service are insufficient to improve alarm fatigue in an intensive care unit: a pilot project. JMIR Hum Factors 2016;3(1):e1.

Nurse–Technology Interactions and Patient Safety

Halley Ruppel, MS, RN*, Marjorie Funk, PhD, RN

KEYWORDS

- Critical care nursing • Technology interactions • Alarm fatigue • Interruptions
- High reliability organizations • Human factors and ergonomics

KEY POINTS

- Nurses are the primary end-users of technology in intensive care units, but nurse–technology interactions receive fragmented attention and can lead to patient safety challenges.
- Nurse–technology interaction includes the input of data into technology and extraction and interpretation of data output, while accounting for the systems in which these processes occur.
- Applying systems-oriented thinking, like high reliability organizations and human factors and ergonomics, has the potential to enhance nurse–technology interactions and improve patient safety.

INTRODUCTION

In intensive care units (ICUs), physiologic monitors, ventilators, and infusion pumps are fixtures at every bedside, and additional complex technology is routinely used to save and prolong lives. Nurses are the end-users of most technology in the ICU, and the ways in which they interact with technology affect quality of care and patient safety. However, little attention is paid to nurse–technology interactions. Nurses rarely receive comprehensive formal education on the use of many of the ubiquitous technologies, and technology is implemented with little consideration for nurses' workflow. Nurses at the bedside are often not given a voice in technology selection; they are instructed to use new devices and find ways to adapt. However, when a new technology is not found to be easy to use or useful, nurses adapt by developing workarounds, or by using the technology ineffectively or inefficiently, at the expense of quality of care.

Disclosure Statement: The authors have nothing to declare.
Yale School of Nursing, 400 West Campus Drive, Orange, CT 06477, USA
* Corresponding author. PO Box 27399, West Haven, CT 06516-7399.
E-mail address: halley.ruppel@yale.edu

Crit Care Nurs Clin N Am 30 (2018) 203–213
https://doi.org/10.1016/j.cnc.2018.02.003
0899-5885/18/© 2018 Elsevier Inc. All rights reserved.

In this article, we explore ICU nurse–technology interactions, past, present and future. We examine:

- The historical relationship between nursing and technology;
- Current challenges related to nurse–technology interactions; and
- Ways in which nurse–technology interactions may be enhanced in the future.

The World Health Organization defines health technology as "the application of organized knowledge and skills in the form of devices, medicines, vaccines, procedures and systems developed to solve a health problem and improve quality of life."[1] Health technology has also been described as a social construct, thus moving it beyond tangible devices and systems.[2] For the purposes of this article, we define health care technology as the information systems, medical devices, hardware, software, and telecommunications used in the provision of health care.

HISTORICAL PERSPECTIVES

In the early and mid-20th century, "physicians thought of nurses much like stethoscopes and surgical instruments, as physical or bodily extensions of physicians."[3(p3)] Nurses were not masters or developers of technology, but technology themselves; they were not taught to interpret data, only to report it. However, as new technology was introduced at an increasingly rapid rate in the second half of the 20th century and hospitalized patients became sicker, nurses, by necessity, were progressively more autonomous in their use of technology and analysis of data.[2]

Still, nurses' unique and critical role in effective use of technology was underappreciated. Fairman and Lynaugh[4] provide the following description of the introduction of cardiac monitors to a general floor at Bethany Hospital in Kansas City, Kansas, in the 1960s, highlighting the pitfalls of an ill-prepared nursing workforce:

> [W]hen Dr. Day introduced cardiac monitors on the general floor, no one taught the nurses about arrhythmias or how to turn off the monitor alarms. Nurses, feeling left out of the process and unable to respond, began to call the physicians at all hours of the day and night when alarms sounded. Shortly thereafter the monitors were removed.[4(p75)]

Even as nurses gained more ownership over the use of technology in hospitals, some nurses sought to distance the profession from technology, criticizing the mechanization of nursing and the disruption of the nurse–patient relationship.[2,3,5] Others saw nurses' growing autonomy over technology as a legitimizing force, one that would bring with it respect for nursing as a profession independent from medicine.[3] Those who embraced technology and those who did not were typically divided between nurses in clinical practice and nurse theorists and educators. Sandelowski[3(p132)] summarizes the issue as "the true nurse, to the frontline nurse, was a doer; the true nurse, according to nurse educators, was a thinker." Although nursing discourse has often held technology at arms length, addressing it with skepticism, nurses at the bedside—especially in ICUs—have had to form intimate relationships with the technologies they use.

CURRENT CHALLENGES RELATED TO NURSE–TECHNOLOGY INTERACTIONS

Nursing's awkward history with technology has created challenges in nurse–technology interactions today. Nursing students receive little formal education on health care technology, but in practice they are often responsible for managing incredibly complex technologies, with the potential to cause harm to the patient if used incorrectly. Most technologies are designed by people unfamiliar with nurses' workflow, and they fail to appreciate the multitude of other devices the nurse is simultaneously managing. Together, these challenges increase patient safety risks and have led to adverse events.

Quantifying adverse events related to nurse–technology interactions is difficult because of the ways in which adverse events are defined and reported. In these reports, medical device-related errors may be user errors or technical failures, and may include errors of other professionals, such as surgeons or anesthesiologists. Still, we know that adverse events are common, costly, and frequently related to medical devices.[6,7] In addition, the ECRI Institute, a nonprofit organization focused on disseminating research about medical devices and products to improve patient safety, produces an annual list of technology hazards. In 2017, many of the top hazards reflected potential breakdowns in nurse–technology interactions (eg, infusion errors, missed alarms, and mistakes in the use of automated medication dispensing cabinets).[8]

Defining Nurse–Technology Interactions

According to the US Food and Drug Administration, the device–user interface includes the size and shape of the device, graphic interfaces, logic of how the device presents information, hardware and accessories, and the packaging and labels.[9] In this article, we conceptualize nurses' interaction with technology as more than the immediate device interface. Nurse–technology interactions also include the processes by which nurses ensure proper input of data into the technology as well as extraction and interpretation of the information output (clinical data, technical data, alarms). Nurses control the input of data by entering patient data, setting goals of care, changing alarm threshold settings, and/or connecting the technology to the patient. Nurses extract output from technology in numerous ways, including performing measurements (eg, thermodilution cardiac output), reviewing and documenting data from multiple screens or sources, and responding to alarms, all in an effort to inform patient care and workflow. The accuracy of nurses' data input into the technology affects the validity and usefulness of data output. In many cases, nurses' interactions with technology also affect patient safety (**Fig. 1**).

For example, to use continuous renal replacement therapy, nurses input patient data (eg, weight), settings for goals of care (eg, flow rates), and may adjust some alarm threshold settings. Nurses also physically set up the device, including ensuring

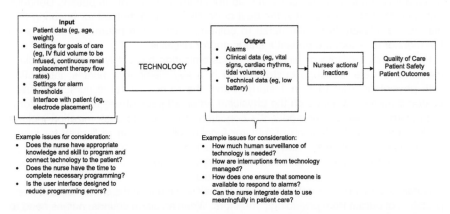

Fig. 1. Schematic diagram of intensive care nurses' interactions with complex technology.

accurate connection of the access and return lines to the patient's catheter. Output from the device includes alarms for values outside set thresholds, as well as clinical data (eg, fluid removal volumes), and technical data (eg, filter pressures). These data are then used by the nurse to inform actions (or inactions) that ultimately influence the quality of care, patient safety, and patient outcomes.

Example: Nurse–Physiologic Monitor Interactions

Challenges arise from all aspects of nurses' interactions with technology (see examples in **Fig. 1**). To highlight the breadth of nurse–technology interaction challenges, we use physiologic monitors as an example and explore select challenges along the continuum of data input, extraction, and interpretation. Although not exhaustive, this exploration of the ways in which nurses interact with physiologic monitors illustrates the complexity of nurse–technology interactions.

Alarms and interruptions

The ways in which nurses input data into technology affects the quality and usefulness of data output from the technology. For physiologic monitors, this process includes ensuring accurate connection to the patient (eg, secure electrode placement, placing the pulse oximeter probe on a well-perfused extremity) and that alarm parameters are appropriately set. In the past several decades, inattention to these processes has contributed to excessive alarms in ICUs and to the development of alarm fatigue.

Although alarms are intended to enhance safety by drawing attention to certain conditions, they have paradoxically become a patient safety risk. Alarms are so often false or nonactionable that nurses consciously or subconsciously ignore or delay their response to them. This phenomenon, called "alarm fatigue," has become a recent high-profile patient safety concern.[10,11] The consequences of alarm fatigue include preventable patient morbidity and mortality when critical true alarms are ignored.[10] By improving input into the monitors, both false and nonactionable alarms can be reduced, subsequently increasing the usefulness of the alarms produced.

False alarms are alarms that are not accurate reflections of the condition indicated. False alarms can be reduced by ensuring good signal quality. Skin preparation before electrode placement may reduce skin impedance and enhance signal quality. Frequent electrode changes have been proposed as a method for reducing false alarms[12]; however, further investigation of this intervention is needed. A more effective solution may be improved electrode technology that can detect electrode failure. Nonactionable alarms are true alarms that do not inform the care of the patient. Because patient conditions vary greatly, the best currently available method for ensuring that alarms are relevant is for the nurse to customize the alarm parameter settings on the monitor to reflect the patient's status and/or baseline.

Factors that facilitate or hinder alarm customization have only been superficially explored to date, although customization is a key element of nurses' interaction with physiologic monitors. In 1 study, within the same unit some nurses reported customizing alarms based on the physician order whereas others reported customizing alarms based on their patient's condition.[13] Barriers to customization include an inadequate understanding of monitor functionality,[14,15] fear of liability for incorrectly customized alarms,[16] and potentially a lack of confidence in nurses' own understanding of the patient condition. Other factors like monitor usability and workload likely also influence nurses' customization of alarms.

Nurse–technology interactions may also break down during the extraction and interpretation of output from physiologic monitors. When an alarm sounds, nurses need to decide whether to interrupt the current task to respond to the alarm. Output needs to be monitored at regular intervals so that clinical trends and changes are not missed, and technical requirements (eg, battery changes) are addressed.

Alarms are by intent interruptive. Interruptions are typically considered to have a negative effect on patient safety, but the ICU workflow may be fundamentally enmeshed with interruptive processes. Interruptions are important insofar as they ensure that critical information reaches the nurse in real time.[17] However, interruptions have been associated with an increased risk of errors.[18] Balancing the inherent nature of interruptions in the ICU with the dangers of interruption presents a system challenge with limited solutions.

Most solutions posed in interruption research have focused on external interruptions from humans (colleagues, patients), rather than interruptions from technology. Some have advocated for a "sterile cockpit" approach to critical tasks, like medication administration, during which interruptions are eliminated.[19,20] Human interrupters can be managed during these tasks with visual indicators; for example, a nurse administering medication can stand in a designated "no interruption zone"[21] or illuminate a "do not disturb" sign outside the room.[22] Interruptions from technology, however, are not amenable to these interventions.

The "sterile cockpit" is logical in the context of aviation, where it originated, because the pilot is responsible for flying 1 plane, so every alarm is relevant to that objective. However, in ICUs, nurses may manage multiple patients, and so they may be interrupted by an alarm that is not relevant to the patient with whom they are currently engaged. When an alarm sounds, it is up to the nurse to determine whether he or she should interrupt the primary task and respond to the alarm, even if this means stopping a critical task.

Monitor watchers and middleware

In an effort to provide appropriate and timely responses to monitor output, rather than increase nurse staffing, hospitals often use technicians to help with technology surveillance. This measure has raised the question of how much human surveillance of technology is needed to maintain patient safety,[23] and how additional personnel can best be used to mediate the nurse–technology interaction.

Monitor watchers or technicians are 1 example of technology surveillance used in many hospitals. They are people whose job it is to watch patient monitors and alert the nurse of potential problems. Nurses often appreciate monitor watchers because they alert nurses to potentially serious events, but many also acknowledge the new challenges to nurse–technology interactions created by adding an intermediary.[24] For example, monitor watchers may not have access to contextual data about the patient, and may, therefore, call the nurse for true but nonactionable alarms. Further research is needed to determine whether patient outcomes are improved by basic surveillance intended to alert nurses to all alarms, or whether skilled surveillance is needed, to be able to interrupt and triage monitor output like rhythms and other waveforms.

Rather than using humans to observe output from physiologic monitors, some hospitals are using secondary notification systems (middleware) to triage alarms by type and escalate alarms when there is no response.[25] Rather than having a monitor watcher call the nurse each time an alarm sounds, middleware sends the alarm to the nurses' pager or cellphone. Decisions about types of alarms forwarded to devices, escalation strategies, and delays can be customized to the unit and programmed into the device.[26] Although the use of middleware for alarm management can be beneficial, it also introduces a new system with which the nurse must interact and has the potential to increase workload if not thoughtfully implemented.

Knowledge and culture

All nurse–technology interactions require that nurses are knowledgeable about the technology and its clinical application. Nurses have been found to have deficient electrocardiographic (ECG) knowledge about factors related to both technology input (eg, electrode placement) and output (eg, rhythm interpretation).[27] In the PULSE trial (Practical Use of the Latest Standards of Electrocardiography),[27] deficient knowledge and practice in ECG monitoring were addressed through an online education intervention, and strategies to implement and sustain change in practice. Although nurses' gains in knowledge were not sustained 15 months after the intervention, improved quality of care related to ECG monitoring was sustained. Improved quality of care included accuracy of electrode placement and rhythm interpretation, as well as the appropriate use of ECG monitoring. Investigators also found that a patient outcome, namely, reduction of in-hospital myocardial infarction, was sustained after the intervention.

The long-term success of the intervention was likely due to the focus on developing ECG monitoring culture changes, not just on enhancing individual nurse knowledge. Indeed, education alone is considered a weak safety intervention,[28] because knowledge decays and because reeducating 1 nurse does not prevent errors by others. Researchers have also found that lack of education is not the most common reason for device-related errors, although retraining the user is often the first solution proposed after an adverse event.[29]

ENHANCING THE FUTURE OF NURSE–TECHNOLOGY INTERACTIONS

Facilitating nurses' safe and efficient use of technology requires consideration for the broader system in which nurses function. Solving problems related to nurse–technology interactions, like alarm fatigue or interruptions, in isolation is necessary but not sufficient. Considering the system in which the nurse–technology interactions occur is critical. Two important concepts from the patient safety literature will help us think more comprehensively about improving nurse–technology interactions in the future: high reliability organizations (HRO) and human factors and ergonomics (HFE).

High Reliability Organizations

The Joint Commission has called for development of HROs to amplify patient safety and quality improvement efforts in health care organizations.[30] They argue that we are failing to make great strides in patient safety because clinicians see "failure as an inevitable feature of their daily work."[30(p463)] In our current system, modest improvements from disparate quality improvement projects are considered to be adequate for improving quality in health care. However, staff develop "project fatigue" from involvement in efforts of limited scope and impact.[30(p459)] In an HRO, however, the organization is universally focused on achieving zero harm, by proactively addressing system weaknesses and developing a workforce that feels individual accountability for the culture of safety and reporting of unsafe conditions.[30]

Today, issues related to nurse–technology interactions are typically addressed through independent quality improvement efforts, with potentially conflicting goals. For example, a workgroup attempting to address the Joint Commission's National Patient Safety Goal on alarm management[31] may try to reduce the use of telemetry monitoring in the organization to decrease alarms. Simultaneously, a workgroup focused on the ECRI recommendation for continuous monitoring of patients receiving opioids[8] may be attempting to increase continuous surveillance monitoring for a subset of patients. If not considered together, these goals could be at odds with one another. Using the concepts of an HRO, a more comprehensive solution to both these problems could be achieved through a reassessment of the whole monitoring process, to clarify indications for monitoring, reduce false and nonactionable alarms from technologies in use, and ensure that all monitoring has appropriate oversight and available staff to respond. As a starting point, organizations should assess all workgroups addressing problems that relate to nurse–technology interactions, and compare their objectives and activities to verify that they are compatible.

Human Factors and Ergonomics

A second concept, HFE, has long been recognized as a mechanism for solving patient safety issues.[32,33] HFE is often thought of as the physical design or interface of devices, but HFE is more than just usability of equipment; it is "designing systems to…improve human performance."[34(p405)] HFE has 3 domains: physical ergonomics, cognitive ergonomics, and macroergonomics.[33] Physical ergonomics refers to the physical aspects of human work and work spaces, such as the location of computers on the unit. Cognitive ergonomics focuses on the cognitive aspects of humans in a system, issues like usability testing of medical devices. Finally, macroergonomics addresses the overall system; for example, how middleware might be used to improve the process of alarm response and decrease response times. The nurse–technology interaction challenges previously discussed, including alarm fatigue and interruptions, are best solved using HFE principles.

One important HFE consideration for nurses' interaction with technology is the integration and interoperability of technologies. Improving nurse–technology interactions in ICUs is hindered by the sheer volume of technology used. Because of the lack of interoperability of the technology, nurses are overburdened with multiple distinct workflows for each technology, and the need to gather data from multiple sources to complete a single task. In a 2008 study,[35] nurses identified integration and interoperability of technology as the most important way to improve workflow, yet 10 years later, single-function technology is being added at an increasingly rapid rate, and the integration of these technologies is slow to materialize.

Visual displays

Not only would interoperability improve nurses' workflow, but integration of data from multiple sources into 1 display can help clinicians to maintain situation awareness.[36,37] Situation awareness is an HFE concept that refers to a person's perception of the environment ("What is going on?"), comprehension of what that means ("So what?"), and projection for what will happen in the future ("Now what?").[30,38,39(p30)] When pieces of patient information are scattered across multiple systems or even multiple screens, clinicians can lose track of information and may lose situation awareness of the patient condition. In their cardiac ICU, Engelman and colleagues[36] developed a graphic display for real-time data from the patient's electronic health record to assist with situation awareness during rounds, which they believe may have contributed to decreased postoperative complications.

Data visualization for clinical information may also enhance situation awareness by improving clinicians' ability to make sense of the vast amounts of data available in health care.[40] In 1 example, Drews and Doig[41] redesigned vital sign displays to better support ICU nurses' work. The new display used visualization tools (eg, trend views) to help nurses interpret patient conditions on average 43% more quickly.[41]

To support nursing practice at the bedside, displays that integrate more than just clinical data may be useful. Koch and colleagues[42] proposed an integrated display that provides not only clinical data about the patient, but also task and systems information to support nurses' workflow. For example, the display could integrate data to facilitate the process of medication administration, including the name of the medication due, location of the medication (eg, refrigerator, patient room, pharmacy), and compatibility with other medications currently infusing.[42] In a study of integrated displays, nurses' situation awareness increased and task completion time decreased.[37] Integrated displays may also help nurses to determine the relevance and validity of alarms by displaying several pieces of information in 1 place, such as recent medication changes along with vital signs.[43]

SUMMARY

Although ICU nurses already consider their work inexorably linked with technology, educators and administrators need to better appreciate this intimate relationship. Technology will continue to pose serious patient safety threats if nurses' interactions with technology are not valued. To achieve better nurse–technology interactions, we need enhanced technology education within prelicensure nursing programs and systems-based HFE approaches to implementing and integrating technology in hospitals.

Nursing as a profession is trying to move away from technically focused education, while simultaneously advocating for recognition as a STEM (science, technology, engineering, and mathematics) profession.[44] Nurses, particularly those starting work in an ICU, find themselves responsible for an abundance of complex technology, but often arrive with little or no education on its design or use. Nurse educators must recognize that understanding and using technology requires not just a technical skill set of knowing which button to push, but rather a rich combination of physiologic knowledge, biomedical engineering principles, and HFE concepts. Nursing will be more readily recognized as a STEM profession if nurses demonstrate authority over the technologies they use, rather than becoming victims of their complexity.

New generations of nurses are often assumed to be more technologically savvy than previous generations, and it may, therefore, be concluded that they need less education on technology use. However, the newest generation of nurses grew up with personal technology that is so user-friendly and intuitive to use, and so inexpensive that it is practically disposable, that they need not actually understand how the technology works. Unlike smart phones, medical devices are not just 1 human–machine interface, but a human–human–machine interface (both the nurse and the patient are end-users of the device).[45] Medical devices are not necessarily designed with the nurse user in mind, and may seem outdated and difficult to use to the new generation of nurses. It may even be harder for new nurses to understand and adapt to technology that seems outdated and inefficient. Including education on health care technology and HFE in prelicensure nursing curricula is more important than ever, so that nurses have the tools to understand and even improve the technology with which they work.

Analogies of health care to aviation often follow traditional professional hierarchical gender roles, equating physicians with pilots. However, in the case of technology use in the ICU, it is more helpful to think of nurses as pilots. The nurse is the most frequent user of the majority of ICU technology, orchestrating technology to achieve care goals and making critical decisions about how and what data to use and bring to the attention of others on the team. Other clinicians often do not know how to use much of the technology at the bedside. That pilots receive extensive simulated training on the use of cockpit technology, and on maintaining situation awareness, seems fundamental. Yet ICU nurses work with similarly complex technology with less interoperability but do not routinely participate in simulation-based technology education. Nurses should receive comprehensive simulation-based training to learn to manage the multitude of devices at the bedside.

Including nurses in usability testing, purchasing decisions, and on data analytics teams will support the development of an HRO, in which nurses perceive their influence over their work environment and patient safety, and are not simply subject to administrative decisions. An HRO would also have a mechanism to understand all technology-related efforts being carried out by the organization, rather than potentially competing efforts from isolated quality improvement initiatives. Additionally, industry is incentivized to show that their devices work and to create new devices sometimes despite what is "needed." Nurses' feedback on how technology is being used, whether it produces meaningful output, and what potential patient safety issues exist are important for taking a proactive approach to value-based care.

In addition to enhanced technology education and better integration of nurses into technology-related administrative decisions, more research is needed to understand nurses' interaction with commonly used technology. Adding personnel like monitor watchers into the process of technology use has the potential to add unnecessary complexity and cost and, as such, requires systematic outcome evaluations. Integrated information displays are a promising mechanism for combining data from multiple devices to support situation awareness and enhancing efficiency of nurses' workflow. Research is needed to understand the cost effectiveness of such devices and the consequence on patient outcomes.

Nurse–technology interactions are a central element of patient safety in ICUs. As technology advances and multiplies, the risk for inefficient and ineffective use of technology and resulting patient safety failures increase. Overhaul of ICU nurses' interactions with bedside technology has the potential to streamline nursing care, reduce costs, and save lives.

REFERENCES

1. World Health Organization (WHO). Technology, health. Health topics n.d. Available at: http://www.who.int/topics/technology_medical/en/.
2. Fairman J. Alternative visions: the nurse-technology relationship in the context of the history of technology. Nurs Hist Rev 1998;6:129–46.
3. Sandelowski M. Devices & desires: gender, technology, and American nursing. Chapel Hill (NC): UNC Press Books; 2000.
4. Fairman J, Lynaugh JE. Critical care nursing: a history. Philadelphia: University of Pennsylvania Press; 2000.
5. Gadow S. Touch and technology: two paradigms of patient care. J Relig Health 1984;23(1):63–9.
6. Pronovost PJ, Thompson DA, Holzmueller CG, et al. Toward learning from patient safety reporting systems. Crit Care 2006;21(4):305–15.
7. Van Den Bos J, Rustagi K, Gray T, et al. The $17.1 billion problem: the annual cost of measurable medical errors. Health Aff 2011;30(4):596–603.
8. ECRI. Top 10 technology hazards for 2017. Available at: www.ecri.org/2017hazards. Accessed March 9, 2018.
9. US Food and Drug Administration (FDA). Applying human factors and usability engineering to medical devices: guidance for industry and Food and Drug Administration staff 2016. Available at: https://www.fda.gov/downloads/MedicalDevices/.../UCM259760.pdf. Accessed March 9, 2018.
10. Joint Commission. Sentinel event alert issue 50: medical device alarm safety in hospitals 2013. Available at: https://www.jointcommission.org/sea_issue_50/.
11. Sendelbach S, Funk M. Alarm fatigue a patient safety concern. AACN Adv Crit Care 2013;24(4):378–86.

12. Cvach MM, Biggs M, Rothwell KJ, et al. Daily electrode change and effect on cardiac monitor alarms: an evidence-based practice approach. J Nurs Care Qual 2013;28(3):265–71.
13. Christensen M, Dodds A, Sauer J, et al. Alarm setting for the critically ill patient: a descriptive pilot survey of nurses' perceptions of current practice in an Australian regional critical care unit. Intensive Crit Care Nurs 2014;30(4):204–10.
14. Gazarian PK, Carrier N, Cohen R, et al. A description of nurses' decision-making in managing electrocardiographic monitor alarms. J Clin Nurs 2015;24(1–2): 151–9.
15. Sowan AK, Tarriela AF, Gomez TM, et al. Nurses' perceptions and practices toward clinical alarms in a transplant cardiac intensive care unit: exploring key issues leading to alarm fatigue. JMIR Hum Factors 2015;2(1):e3.
16. Honan L, Funk M, Maynard M, et al. Nurses' perspectives on clinical alarms. Am J Crit Care 2015;24(5):387–95.
17. Rivera-Rodriguez A, Karsh B-T. Interruptions and distractions in healthcare: review and reappraisal. Qual Saf Health Care 2010;19(4):304–12.
18. Westbrook JI, Woods A, Rob MI, et al. Association of interruptions with an increased risk and severity of medication administration errors. Arch Intern Med 2010;170(8):683–90.
19. Hohenhaus SM, Powell SM. Distractions and interruptions: development of a healthcare sterile cockpit. Newborn Infant Nurse Rev 2008;8(2):108–10.
20. Kapur N, Parand A, Soukup T, et al. Aviation and healthcare: a comparative review with implications for patient safety. JRSM Open 2015;7(1). 2054270415616548.
21. Anthony K, Wiencek C, Bauer C, et al. No interruptions please: impact of a no interruption zone on medication safety in intensive care units. Crit Care Nurse 2010;30(3):21–9.
22. Sasangohar F, Donmez B, Easty AC, et al. Mitigating nonurgent interruptions during high-severity intensive care unit tasks using a task-severity awareness tool: a quasi-controlled observational study. Crit Care 2015;30(5):1150.e1-6.
23. Funk M. As health care technology advances: benefits and risks. Am J Crit Care 2011;20(4):285–91.
24. Funk M, Ruppel H, Blake N, et al. Use of monitor watchers in hospitals: characteristics, training, and practices. Biomed Instrum Technol 2016;50(6):428–38.
25. Cvach MM, Frank RJ, Doyle P, et al. Use of pagers with an alarm escalation system to reduce cardiac monitor alarm signals. J Nurs Care Qual 2014;29(1):9–18.
26. Jacques S. Factors that affect design of secondary alarm notification systems. Biomed Instrum Technol 2017;51(s2):16–20.
27. Funk M, Fennie KP, Stephens KE, et al. Association of implementation of practice standards for electrocardiographic monitoring with nurses' knowledge, quality of care, and patient outcomes. Circ Cardiovasc Qual Outcomes 2017;10(2): e003132.
28. Pronovost PJ, Goeschel CA, Olsen KL, et al. Reducing health care hazards: lessons from the commercial aviation safety team. Health Aff 2009;28:w479–89.
29. Johnson TR, Tang X, Graham MJ, et al. Attitudes toward medical device use errors and the prevention of adverse events. Jt Comm J Qual Patient Saf 2007; 33(11):689–94.
30. Chassin MR, Loeb JM. High-reliability health care: getting there from here. Milbank Q 2013;91(3):459–90.
31. Joint Commission on Accreditation of Healthcare Organizations. The Joint Commission announces 2014 national patient safety goal. Jt Comm Perspect 2013; 33(7):1, 3–4.

32. Carayon P, Wetterneck TB, Rivera-Rodriguez AJ, et al. Human factors systems approach to healthcare quality and patient safety. Appl Ergon 2014;45(1):14–25.
33. Gurses AP, Ozok AA, Pronovost PJ. Time to accelerate integration of human factors and ergonomics in patient safety. BMJ Qual Saf 2012;21(4):347–51.
34. Harder KA, Marc D. Human factors issues in the intensive care unit. AACN Adv Crit Care 2013;24(4):405–14.
35. Bolton LB, Gassert CA, Cipriano PF. Smart technology, enduring solutions. Health Inf Manag 2008;22(4):24–30.
36. Engelman D, Higgins TL, Talati R, et al. Maintaining situational awareness in a cardiac intensive care unit. J Thorac Cardiovasc Surg 2014;147(3):1105–6.
37. Koch SH, Weir C, Westenskow D, et al. Evaluation of the effect of information integration in displays for ICU nurses on situation awareness and task completion time: a prospective randomized controlled study. Int J Med Inform 2013;82(8): 665–75.
38. Endsley MR. Toward a theory of situation awareness in dynamic systems. Hum Factors 1995;37(1):32–64.
39. Flin R, Winter J, Sarac C, et al, World Health Organization. Human factors in patient safety: review of topics and tools. Geneva (Switzerland): World Health Organization; 2009. p. 2.
40. Wanderer JP, Nelson SE, Ehrenfeld JM, et al. Clinical data visualization: the current state and future needs. J Med Syst 2016;40(12):275.
41. Drews FA, Doig A. Evaluation of a configural vital signs display for intensive care unit nurses. Hum Factors 2014;56(3):569–80.
42. Koch SH, Weir C, Haar M, et al. Intensive care unit nurses' information needs and recommendations for integrated displays to improve nurses' situation awareness. J Am Med Inform Assoc 2012;19(4):583–90.
43. Egan M. Clinical dashboards: impact on workflow, care quality, and patient safety. Crit Care Nurs Q 2006;29(4):354–61.
44. Hassmiller SB, Mensik JS. The power of ten: a conversational approach to tackling the top ten priorities in nursing. Indianapolis (IN): Sigma Theta Tau; 2016.
45. McConnell EA. The impact of machines on the work of critical care nurses. Crit Care Nurs Q 1990;12(4):45–52.

Intravenous Smart Pumps

Usability Issues, Intravenous Medication Administration Error, and Patient Safety

Karen K. Giuliano, PhD, RN, MBA[a,b,*]

KEYWORDS

- IV infusion/medication error • IV smart pump • Patient safety
- Medical device usability

KEY POINTS

- Although the use of intravenous smart pumps has been associated with reductions in medication error rates, they have not eliminated error.
- Current data do not support that the use of intravenous smart pumps has had a measurable impact on decreasing adverse drug events.
- The administration of multiple intravenous infusions, secondary infusions, intravenous boluses, and titrated doses are particularly prone to errors.
- Intravenous smart pump programming errors often result from use errors related to the infusion device interface.
- There is a clear need for innovation in intravenous smart pumps to address usability and safety challenges.

INTRODUCTION

Intravenous (IV) infusion pump systems are among the most frequently used technologies in health care. An estimated 90% of hospital patients receive IV medications via infusion pumps,[1] an indication of how pervasive these devices are in patient care, particularly in critical and acute care settings. Clinical use of IV smart pumps with built-in dose error reduction systems (DERS) began at Massachusetts General Hospital in 1996 and has since become widely accepted as a standard of care for the reduction of infusion-related medication error.[2] A 2012 national survey by the American Society of Healthcare System Pharmacists found a 77% adoption rate of IV Smart

Disclosure: The author has performed consulting services for Ivenix.
[a] Northeastern University, 360 Huntington Avenue, Boston, MA 02115, USA; [b] The Center for Nursing Research and Advanced Nursing Practice, Orlando Regional Medical Center, Orlando, FL, USA
* Corresponding author. Massachusetts General Hospital, Yvonne L. Munn Center for Nursing Research, 360 Huntington Avenue, Boston, MA 02115.
E-mail address: kkgiuliano96@gmail.com

Crit Care Nurs Clin N Am 30 (2018) 215–224
https://doi.org/10.1016/j.cnc.2018.02.004   ccnursing.theclinics.com
0899-5885/18/© 2018 The Author. Published by Elsevier Inc. This is an open access article under the
CC BY-NC-ND license (http://creativecommons.org/licenses/by-nc-nd/4.0/).

pumps by US hospitals.[3] Although the use of IV smart pumps has been associated with decreases in medication error rates, they have not eliminated error.[4–6] Furthermore, current data do not support that the use of IV smart pumps has had a measurable impact on decreasing adverse drug events (ADEs).[4,7,8]

Common sources of user error include overriding dose error alerts and, even more concerning, manually bypassing the drug libraries and DERS completely.[9,10] The complexity of the device user interface, the time required to program the DERS, and incomplete drug libraries are among the most frequently cited reasons that nurses bypass IV smart pump safety features.[11] The complexity of IV medication administration and the multiple steps involved demands close attention to detail and ultimately relies heavily on human–device interaction to detect and mitigate errors. Clinicians in the busy critical care and medical-surgical clinical environments are frequently interrupted and rushed during IV smart pump programming. As a result, the overriding of alerts and programming outside of the DERS owing to time constraints and competing work demands are recognized as a part of daily clinical practice.[9,12–15] Despite an increasing focus in health care on patient safety and quality of care, and despite improvements in technology, medication errors and usability issues with IV smart pumps are a significant patient safety issue.[16] A recent review of the US Food and Drug Administration (FDA) Manufacturer and User Device Experience database for 2015 to 2017 revealed more than 23,000 submitted reports of malfunction and injury for the 3 most commonly used large volume IV smart pumps (Alaris, Baxter, and Hospira).

The ubiquity of IV smart pumps, along with a sense of urgency to address IV medication safety, has garnered the attention of several organizations focused on patient safety. The Association for the Advancement of Medical Instrumentation (AAMI) and the FDA cosponsored a summit in 2010 to prioritize patient safety related to IV infusions as a national concern.[17] In 2012, the National Quality Forum conducted an environmental analysis that resulted in 13 recommendations to improve safety of IV infusion devices.[12] The 2014 Emergency Care Research Institute identified alarm hazards and infusion pump medication errors as priorities that need immediate attention.[18] In 2015, Association for the Advancement of Medical Instrumentation initiated a multiyear national coalition to address IV infusion device safety.

OVERVIEW: INTRAVENOUS INFUSION ERROR

IV medication administration is a complex, multistep process that provides numerous opportunities for error, with administration at the point of care as the part of the process most vulnerable to errors.[19,20] Medication error is a general phrase that encompasses multiple and distinct ways in which IV infusions can go wrong at virtually every stage of the medication delivery process. A failure modes and effects analysis of the set of processes used to deliver continuous drug infusions at an 11-bed pediatric ICU identified 6 elements of the process: (1) selecting the drug, (2) selecting a dose, (3) selecting an infusion rate, (4) calculating and ordering the infusion, (5) programming the infusion pump, and (6) delivering the infusion. The last 3 elements of the process had the highest risk profiles.[21]

Table 1 provides an example that outlines and compares the required steps for programming a normal saline infusion at 125 mL/h within the medical-surgical drug library on 3 widely used large-volume IV smart pumps: BD/Alaris, Baxter Sigma, and Hospira Plum A+. These 3 manufacturers represent approximately 88% of the large-volume IV smart pumps in current clinical use in US hospitals, with Alaris as the most widely used.[22] Each pump requires between 11 and 17 steps to program an normal saline infusion, making it easy to see that even low risk infusions are not simple to program.

Table 1		
Required steps for programming an NS infusion within the M/S drug library on the Alaris, Baxter, and Hospira Plum A+ IV smart pumps		
Step	Sigma (SW Version v6.02.07)	Alaris (SW Version 9.19)	Plum A+ (SW Version 13.41.00.002)
1	Push "ON" button	Push "ON" button	Push "ON" button
2	New patient? Hit YES	New patient? Hit YES	New patient? Hit YES
3	Brings up library list, use arrow key to choose M/S library	Displays profile used last. Hit NO	Brings up library list, use arrow key to choose M/S library
4	OK	Brings up drug library list, select M/S library	ENTER
5	Enter IV	CONFIRM	Hit Arrow up "A"
6	Use arrow to scroll down to IV Fluids	Asks for patient ID, Hit EXIT	Arrow/Page down to IV Fluids
7	OK	Brings up list of available channels (up to 4), select channel	ENTER
8	Choose PRIMARY or SECONDARY	Chose from Guardrails drugs, Guardrails IV fluids, or basic, Chose IV FLUIDS	Enter RATE
9	OK	Select alphabet range that includes the letter "N"	Hit ARROW DOWN BUTTON
10	Enter RATE	Select the letter "N"	Enter VTBI
11	OK	Select NS	Hit START
12	Enter VTBI	Correct? Hit YES	
13	OK	Hit RATE ARROW KEY	
14	Confirm volume given as 0	Enter rate using keypad	
15	Hit RUN	Hit arrow key to chose VTBI	
16		Enter VTBI	
17		Hit START	

Abbreviations: IV, intravenous; M/S, medical-surgical; NS, normal saline; VTBI, volume to be infused.

An analysis by the Emergency Care Research Institute patient safety organization of medication errors at 80 health care organizations—including acute care and pediatric hospitals and long-term care facilities—categorized the medication use process as having 4 stages, or "nodes": prescribing, dispensing, administering, and monitoring. Of 695 ADE submitted by participating health care organizations over a 5-week period in 2011, the majority (67.7%) occurred during medication administration, followed by dispensing (16.1%), prescribing (8.5%), and monitoring (7.8%). IV-related errors, the most frequent occurrences of medication errors reported, represented 36.9% of administration-only ADE reported in this analysis. Some ADE involved errors at multiple stages of the process. The most commonly reported types of IV administration errors included drug not given (22.9%), due to failure to open the tubing (especially when a secondary infusion was administered) or to connect the IV line to the patient to allow the drug to be infused; wrong pump rate (20.3%); wrong drug (16.9%); and wrong dose (13.6%).[20]

Programming errors are known to contribute to medication errors involving IV infusion devices, because data support that the majority of ADE are the result of incorrect programming.[12] Examples of programming errors include incorrectly entering (or selecting from menus of) drug names, doses/concentrations, rates, and times[23]; bypassing the drug library (either accidentally or intentionally)[7]; and administering an incorrect or unauthorized medication, and overriding drug limits or alerts.[7] Programming errors can result from incorrect clinical decisions, mental computation errors, keystroke errors, or use errors related to the infusion device interface (eg, entering information into the wrong field).[24]

ERROR PRONE PROGRAMMING TASKS: MULTIPLE INFUSIONS, SECONDARY INFUSIONS, AND BOLUS DOSING

Administration of multiple IV infusions, secondary infusions, IV bolus, and titrated doses are particularly prone to errors. Landmark studies by the University Health Network in Toronto[25,26] examined the types of reported incidents and errors associated with both sequential infusions through the same channel of a single infusion pump and concurrent infusions using separate channels on the same IV pump or on multiple pumps. Incidents reported and analyzed from the Institute for Safe Medical Practices in Canada for almost a decade (May 2000 to April 2010) indicated that incidents occurred during all methods of multiple IV infusion administration—sequential, concurrent, or a combination of both. Given that some patients can receive as many as 10 to 15 IV infusions at 1 time,[26] via different methods of administration and multiple pumps and lines, the potential for mix-ups and errors is very real. Multiple infusions place additional cognitive demands on clinicians, are not well-standardized, have many associated failure modes, and errors are not easily detected.[25]

Medication administration by secondary infusion is the most common method for administering IV medications ordered for 1-time or intermittent dosing, especially IV antibiotics. Secondary administration is designed to allow the primary continuous infusion to resume automatically once the secondary infusion is completes. To ensure that the secondary medication infuses as intended, most IV smart pumps (with the exception of the Hospira Plum series) require the nurse to manually increase the secondary IV bag height, so that the secondary hydrostatic pressure differential is great enough to prevent flow of the primary infusion until the secondary infuses completely. If the bag height differential is not great enough to prevent flow of the primary infusion, the secondary may not infuse at all, or both bags may infuse concurrently at unpredictable rates. This will occur even if the pump is programmed correctly.[25] Either situation leads to a medication administration error that is rarely identified or reported. The need for bag height differential for most IV infusion pumps, the complex acute care environment, the high cognitive load required for IV medication administration, a high frequency of interruptions, and a lack of standardized training and education regarding the relevant principles for secondary infusions all contribute to increased human error during secondary medication administration.[25]

During their field study, Cassano-Piché and colleagues[25] identified the following issues related to secondary infusion as having the potential to lead directly to patient harm: secondary medication is connected to a high-alert primary medication infusion; secondary medication is a continuous infusion of a high-alert medication; insufficient bag head height differential between primary and secondary infusions; secondary tubing is connected to the wrong port along the primary tubing; secondary IV tubing remains clamped after the secondary infusion has started; the secondary IV tubing is connected to a primary infusion set with no back check valve; and the infusion pump does not support the administration of a secondary infusion on a primary line programmed using the drug library. The following case study on error with secondary infusion was included in their report:

> *An experienced nurse worked on a general ward that rarely ran secondary infusions. She was not trained specifically on this feature of the infusion pump, but was able to figure out how to use it. Her patient was receiving D5W mixed with half-normal saline via an infusion pump at 40 mL/h. She had orders to administer morphine prepared in a 100 mL bag. She administered it as a secondary infusion on the D5W– half-saline primary line at a rate of 2 mL/h. The nurse was caring for several other patients and wanted to receive an alert after 5 hours to check on the morphine infusion before the end of her shift, so she (deliberately) set the volume to be infused (VTBI) to 10 mL instead of the 100 mL bag volume, expecting the pump to stop and sound a volume-complete alarm, as it does in the primary mode. However, the secondary mode is not designed this way on all pumps. After 5 hours, the pump automatically switched from the secondary to the primary mode, resulting in the remaining 90 mL of morphine in the secondary bag being infused at 40 mL/h. The nurse went home at the end of her shift not having noticed the error, and several hours later the patient was found dead in bed.[25(p35)]*

As a single dose of medication administered in a short period of time for a therapeutic purpose, medication administration by IV bolus dosing has the potential to cause more serious harm to patients than infusions administered at slower rates. In an observational study of IV medication preparation and administration in an ICU of a teaching hospital, the most common type of error was the injection of bolus doses faster than the recommended rate.[27] In another observational study of IV medication administration in 6 wards across 2 teaching hospitals, administration by bolus was associated with a 312% increased risk of error.[28]

Cassano-Piché and colleagues[25] observed 3 methods that were used for IV bolus dosing when not using the IV smart pump bolus feature: temporarily increasing the rate of a currently infusing medication, preparing an IV syringe with the bolus dose and administering the bolus as a manual IV push, and preparing an IV bag with the bolus and administering the bolus as a secondary infusion. Of the 3, only the latter two were considered safe.[25] It is important to note that regardless of which method is used, the dead volume contained in the primary infusion tubing will be flushed as the bolus is administered, making it unsafe to use any method of IV bolus dosing in an IV line, which contains high-alert medications.

Issues identified as contributing to error with IV bolus dosing on IV smart pumps included IV smart pump does not have a bolus feature, the bolus feature may not be enabled for every relevant medication, a lack of familiarity with programming the bolus, and complexity of the bolus feature leading to excessive amounts of time required to execute the programming sequence.[25] Additionally, the FDA recall database includes several class I recalls related to bolus features and functionality. The following case study provides an example of why it is unsafe to administer IV bolus doses using temporary primary infusion rate increases[25]:

> *During a shadowing session, a nurse described a past incident during which she was administering a bolus by programming the primary infusion to run at the fastest possible rate. She intended to specify a VTBI to limit the bolus; however, she became distracted by a patient across the hall who was self-extubating. She pressed the start button without changing the VTBI from the previously programmed value (entire bag volume); while she was assisting the patient across the hall, the first patient received a very large dose of morphine. The patient was not seriously harmed, but the nurse was so upset*

that she no longer administers bolus infusions by changing the primary infusion rate.[25(p71)]

USABILITY ISSUES AND CLINICAL USE

As illustrated by the previous examples, medication errors should be considered failures in the drug delivery system, not human errors by front-line staff.[21] The 2010 Association for the Advancement of Medical Instrumentation/FDA summit on infusion device called for mitigating use errors with infusion devices by developing "design safety features that make it easy for the user to do the right thing."[17] In a presummit survey, clinical, pharmaceutical, engineering, academic, and regulatory professionals identified a number of usability and user interface challenges with infusion devices, among many other challenges. Examples of the most troublesome issues cited by summit participants included the following.

- Programming features that require multiple screens to properly program devices, pushing of several buttons for programming, and pumps that are "incredibly difficult to program."
- Confusing software menus and selection keys, and the use of numeric key pads, which result in "predictable" data entry errors.
- Screens that are difficult to read and that are at improper heights.
- Devices that are too big and too heavy, and that must be moved from IV pole to IV pole when patients are in transit.

In busy, stressful clinical settings, usability challenges contribute to IV medication errors, even by highly experienced clinicians.[11,29] Usability issues are compounded when multiple devices, and different brands of devices are in use. To safely deliver IV medication using multiple infusion devices, clinicians are required to master different pumps, different user interfaces, different accessories and supplies, and distinguish the most appropriate time for each to be used. A single patient can receive multiple infusions from different devices at the same time, and a single clinician can work in multiple settings of care. Variations in the standards of care for IV infusion therapy, different patient populations, transitions in care, and different environments of care can also increase the potential for error.[15]

HUMAN FACTORS DESIGN AND INTRAVENOUS SMART PUMP USABILITY

The FDA has been advocating for the inclusion of human factors engineering as part of the medical device design process since the release of their guidance document in 2000.[30] The FDA now requires that potential hazards related to medical device use be addressed during device development, with user testing as the foundation at each stage of the product development process. Ongoing documentation of these efforts and adequate mitigation of all identified risks is now required as part of the regulatory approval process. The goal is to minimize use-related hazards, and to ensure that users are able to use medical devices safely and effectively in the environment for which they are intended.[30] Although these requirements exist for any new devices being introduced into the market, most of these requirements did not exist when some of the infusion devices in current clinical use were first introduced.

Over the past decade, the safety and usability challenges associated with IV smart pumps have resulted in numerous FDA recalls. When recalls occur, they are classified by the FDA into 1 of 3 possible classes according to the degree of associated health hazard.

Class I: a situation in which there is a reasonable probability that the use of, or exposure to, a violative product will cause serious adverse health consequences or death.

Class II: a situation in which use of, or exposure to, a violative product may cause temporary or medically reversible adverse health consequences or where the probability of serious adverse health consequences is remote.

Class III: a situation in which use of, or exposure to, a violative product is not likely to cause adverse health consequences.

A review of the FDA recall database for large volume IV smart pumps between the dates of January 1, 2015, and October 9, 2017, revealed a total of 37 recalls of large volume IV infusion pumps, tubing and/or software for Alaris, Baxter and Hospira. Five of these recalls (14%) were class (**Table 2**).[31]

Table 2
FDA recalls for large volume IV infusion pumps, tubing and/or software for Alaris, Baxter and Hospira between the dates of January 1, 2015 and October 9, 2017

	Total	Class 1	Class 2	Class 3
Alaris	17	4	13	0
Baxter	8	1	7	0
Hospira	12	0	12	0

Additionally, 2 highly publicized recalls resulted in IV smart pumps being permanently removed from the market. In 2010, the Baxter Colleague was discontinued. The FDA gave Baxter 2 years to complete their recall of between 200,000 and 250,000 IV smart pump channels in the US health care market. Customers were given the opportunity to transition to the Baxter Sigma IV Smart Pump, or receive a refund.[32]

In 2015 after multiple recalls, the Hospira Symbiq was permanently discontinued for sale. Because infusion devices are potentially life-saving, removing them from clinical use cannot happen immediately. It requires planning and a sequential approach. Unfortunately, shortly after the Symbiq was discontinued for sale, the FDA, the US Department of Homeland Security's Industrial Control Systems Cyber Emergency Response Team, and Hospira became aware of cybersecurity vulnerabilities associated with the Symbiq Infusion System. Hospira and an independent researcher confirmed that Hospira's Symbiq Infusion System could be accessed remotely through a hospital's network, allowing an unauthorized user to control the device and alter IV medication infusions. Although the FDA and Hospira were not aware of any ADE or unauthorized access, the Symbiq Infusion System removal needed to be accelerated to mitigate for this very serious risk.[33]

NEED FOR INNOVATION

According to Nathaniel Sims, a well-known inventor and creator of the DERS, a broad view of the future of innovation in IV smart pumps would include[34]:

- Elimination of manual order entry and transcription;
- Patient-aware clinical support;
- Assisted caregiver programming;

- Autoprogramming, in which medication orders are sent directly to the infusion pump from a verified provider or pharmacy information system and then confirmed by a clinician before an infusion is administered;
- Autodocumentation of infusion pump programming, status, and alerts in electronic information systems; and
- Enhanced alerts and second checks.

An infusion pump workshop convened by the Applied Physics Laboratory at Johns Hopkins University in 2012 focused on a systems engineering approach to human factors solutions to most effectively address usability challenges.[35] Specifically, workshop participants cited the need for improvements in:

- System integration at the health information technology level—for ordering, pharmacy supply and control, documentation, and adherence to safety control—and at the bedside level for pumps and accessories;
- Programming navigation with better designed user interfaces;
- Information presentation and prioritization, with better ergonomics and visual and audio displays of critical information;
- Control standardization to minimize confusion and variation of controls and function representation on products from different pump manufacturers; and
- Context awareness, with information about all pumps, IV bags, and drugs for a single patient to provide a more comprehensive look at a patient's condition.

Finally, a review by Giuliano and Neimi (2015) lists several additional innovation needs[16]:

- Current pumps have a limited ability to communicate with one another.
- Pumps need to provide cross-pump guidance for the entire patient therapy.
- Pumps typically do not make use of patient information on the health care enterprise, making patient-centered guidance virtually impossible.
- Interoperability with other systems that provide pertinent patient-specific information (such as physiologic and laboratory parameters) that allows for profile-based and seamless patient care management is needed.
- Autoprogramming is ideal but, until those capabilities are more widely available, manual programming must be simplified. Most pumps are manually programmed through a series of nonobvious button pushes, do not use touchscreen technology, and the navigation to the DERS is often difficult and time consuming.
- The visibility of screens must be improved. Because of a small screen size and the limited capabilities of the pump, users are not able to see information to support optimal infusion delivery.
- Devices should be lighter, smaller, more portable, more rugged, and usable at eye level. Most pumps today are large, heavy, and not designed with transportability in mind.

SUMMARY

There is a clear need for innovation in IV smart pumps to address usability and safety challenges. Although it is possible to address some of the issues with changes in clinical processes, the most fundamental challenges need to be addressed through innovation and the development of new technology using a human factors approach. As the primary users of the most complex configurations of IV infusion devices, critical care nurses are in the key position to guide innovation and conduct outcomes research to measure the impact of innovation in this very important area of patient safety.

REFERENCES

1. Husch M, Sullivan C, Rooney D. Insights from the sharp end of intravenous medication errors: implications for infusion pump technology. Qual Saf Health Care 2005;14(2):80–6.
2. Giuliano KK, Ruppel H. Are smart pumps smart enough? Nursing 2017;47(3): 64–6.
3. Pederson CA, Schneider PJ, Scheckelhoff DJ. ASHP national survey of pharmacy practice in hospital settings: monitoring and patient education-2012. Am J Health Syst Pharm 2013;70(9):787–803.
4. Ohashi K, Dalleur O, Dykes PC, et al. Benefits and risks of using smart pumps to reduce medication error rates: a systematic review. Drug Saf 2014;37(12): 1011–20.
5. Hertzel C, Sousa VD. The use of smart pumps for preventing medication errors. J Infus Nurs 2009;32(5):257–67.
6. Murdoch LJ, Cameron VL. Smart infusion technology: a minimum safety standard for intensive care? Br J Nurs 2008;17(10):630–6.
7. Rothschild JM, Keohane CA, Cook EF, et al. A controlled trial of smart infusion pumps to improve medication safety in critically ill patients. Crit Care Med 2005;33(3):533–40.
8. Nuckols TK, Bower AG, Paddock SM, et al. Programmable infusion pumps in ICUs: an analysis of corresponding adverse drug events. J Gen Intern Med 2008;23(1):41–5.
9. McAlearney AS, Chisolm DJ, Schweikhart S, et al. The story behind the story: physician skepticism about relying on clinical information technologies to reduce medical errors. Int J Med Inform 2007;76(11–12):836–42.
10. Kirkbridge G, Vermace B. Smart pumps: implications for nurse leaders. Nurs Adm Q 2011;35(2):110–8.
11. Carayon P, Hundt AS, Wetterneck TB. Nurses' acceptance of Smart IV pump technology. Int J Med Inform 2010;79(6):401–11.
12. National Quality Forum. Critical paths for creating data platforms: intravenous infusion pump devices. Washington, DC: National Quality Forum; 2012.
13. Campoe KR, Giuliano KK. Impact of frequent interruption on nurses' patient-controlled analgesia programming performance. Hum Factors 2017;59(8): 1204–13.
14. Westbrook JI, Woods A, Rob MI, et al. Association of interruptions with an increased risk and severity of medication administration errors. Arch Intern Med 2010;170(8):683–90.
15. Giuliano KK, Su WT, Degnan DD, et al. Intravenous smart pump drug library compliance: a descriptive study of 44 hospitals. J Patient Saf 2017. [Epub ahead of print].
16. Giuliano KK, Niemi C. The urgent need for innovation in IV smart pumps. Nurs Manage 2015;46(3):17–9.
17. Association for the Advancement of Medical Instrumentation (AAMI). Infusing patients safely. Priority issues from the AAMI/FDA infusion device summit. 2010. p. 1–48.
18. Emergency Care Research Institute (ECRI). Top 10 health hazards for 2015. Plymouth (PA): Health Devices; 2014. p. 1–33.

19. Maddox RR, Danello S, Williams CK, et al. Intravenous infusion safety initiative: collaboration, evidence-based best practices, and "smart" technology help avert high-risk adverse drug events and improve patient outcomes. Rockville (MD): Agency for Healthcare Research and Quality; 2008. p. 1–14.
20. Huber C, Rebold B, Wallace C. ERCI institute PSO deep Dive™ analyzes medication events. Plymouth (PA): ECRI Institute; 2012.
21. Apkon M, Leonard J, Probst L. Design of a safer approach to IV drug infusions: failure mode effect analysis. Qual Saf Health Care 2004;13:265–71.
22. Edge J. Infusion Pumps Report 2015. Infusion pumps and accessories - World. Englewood (CO): IHS; 2013.
23. Keohane CA, Hayes J, Saniuk C. Intravenous medication safety and smart infusion systems: lessons learned and future opportunities. J Infus Nurs 2005; 28(5):321–8.
24. Rayo M, Smith P, Weinger MB. Assessing medication safety technology in the intensive care unit. Proceedings of the Human Factors and Ergonomics Society 51st Annual Meeting. Baltimore, October 1–5, 2007.
25. Cassano-Piché A, Fan M, Sabovitch S, et al. Multiple intravenous infusions phase 1b: practice and training scan. Ont Health Technol Assess Ser 2012;12(16):1.
26. Easty T, Cassano-Piché A, White R. Multiple intravenous infusions phase 1a: situation scan summary report. Toronto (CA): Health Technology Safety Research Team, University Health Network; 2010.
27. Fahimi F, Ariapanah P, Faizi M, et al. Errors in preparation and administration of intravenous medications in the intensive care unit of a teaching hospital: an observational study. Aust Crit Care 2008;21(2):110–6.
28. Westbrook JI, Rob MI, Woods A, et al. Errors in the administration of intravenous medications in hospital and the role of correct procedures and nurse experience. BMJ Qual Saf 2011;20(12):1027–34.
29. Carayon P, Wetterneck TB, Rivera-Rodriguez AJ, et al. Human factors systems approach to healthcare quality and patient safety. Appl Ergon 2014;45(1):14–25.
30. Kaye R, Crowley J. Medical device use-safety: incorporating human factors engineering into risk management. Silver Spring (MD): FDA; 2000.
31. US Food and Drug Administration (FDA). Medical device recalls. 2017. Available at: https://www.accessdata.fds.gov/scripts/cdrh/cfdocs/cfRES/res.cfm. Accessed October 9, 2017.
32. Kamp J. Baxter to replace or pay refunds on drug pumps. Wall St J 2010. Available at: https://www.wsj.com/articles/SB10001424052748704518904575365242953771732. Accessed October 20, 2015.
33. US Food and Drug Administration (FDA). Symbiq Infusion System by Hospira: FDA Safety Communication - Cybersecurity Vulnerabilities. 2015. Available at: https://www.fda.gov/safety/medwatch/safetyinformation/safetyalertsforhuman medicalproducts/ucm456832.htm. Accessed October 20, 2015.
34. Sims NM, Schneider DI. What you can do now interim: technology applications to help achieve IV-IT interoperability. Biomed Instrum Technol 2012;46(5):345–9.
35. Ravitz A. Improving safety of medication infusion pump through simulation and applying systems engineering principles and best practices. Baltimore (MD): Johns Hopkins; 2014.

Human Factors in Medical Device Design
Methods, Principles, and Guidelines

Russell J. Branaghan, PhD

KEYWORDS

- Intensive care unit • Human factors • Adverse events • Medical devices • Usability

KEY POINTS

- A total of 400,000 to 500,000 patients die in intensive care units (ICUs) each year, largely because ICUs care for the sickest patients.
- On the other hand, factors such as workload, shift changes, handoffs, alarm fatigue, inadequate team communication, and difficult-to-use medical devices contribute to the problem.
- This article focuses on the human factors of those medical devices, a significant cause of adverse events in the ICU.

INTRODUCTION

There are approximately 6000 intensive care units (ICUs) across the United States,[1] caring for nearly 55,000 patients every day.[2] This accounts for approximately 10% of all hospital beds and 1.5% of US gross national product,[3] numbers that will only increase as the population ages.

More important, 400,000 to 500,000 patients die in ICUs each year,[1] largely because ICUs care for the sickest patients. On the other hand, factors such as workload, shift changes, handoffs, alarm fatigue, inadequate team communication, and difficult-to-use medical devices contribute to the problem. For example, Donchin and colleagues[4] estimate 1.7 errors per patient per day in ICUs, with 29% of these errors having potential to cause significant harm or death. This article focuses on the human factors (HF) of those medical devices, a significant cause of adverse events in the ICU.[5]

HUMAN FACTORS

The most complex part of any medical device is the person using it. Unless the device operates entirely on its own, the user's behavior, capabilities, and limitations

Disclosure Statement: The author has nothing to disclose.
Human Systems Engineering Program, Ira A. Fulton Schools of Engineering, Arizona State University, 7271 East Sonoran Arroyo Mall, 150 J Santa Catalina Hall, Mesa, AZ 88001, USA
E-mail address: Russell.Branaghan@asu.edu

are key to its effectiveness and safety. HF applies scientific knowledge about human behavior, capabilities, and limitations to design.[6] By understanding how humans think, decide, and act under stress, we can engineer products that humans can use safely, correctly, and reliably.[7] Because people are complex and multifaceted, HF includes practitioners from cognitive psychology, sociology, anthropology, industrial engineering, industrial design, medicine and related health sciences, biomechanics, and more. The common denominator is that each focuses on human behavior, capabilities, and limitations. This focus not only improves the performance and satisfaction of health care providers, but also improves patient safety.

It is also important to describe what HF is not, articulated by Lee and colleagues[6] who point out that HF is not simply applying a checklist to determine if a product is easy to use. The variability of people, situations, tasks, technologies, and environments make creation of such a checklist impossible. Second, HF is not simply using oneself as a model of the end user. There are sizable person-to-person variations in size, strength, reading ability, stress, exhaustion, technical sophistication, and so on. This requires design for a wide range of users, rather than just one "type." Unfortunately, organizations may believe that good HF is easy or "common sense," but if that were true, the world would be chock full of easy-to-use medical devices. Personal experiences of health care providers, as well as numerous product recalls and adverse events, suggest quite the opposite.

USABILITY

Usability[8] is a term so closely related to HF that it is often treated as a synonym. Rubin and Chisnell[9] argue that "a usable product enables users to do what they want to do, in the way they expect to be able to do it, without hindrance or questions." Usability is defined along 5 dimensions.

- *Learnability* refers to users' ability to begin using a new system quickly and correctly, and to develop proficiency within a reasonable time frame.
- *Efficiency* refers to whether the system allows users to complete tasks more easily than working without the product.
- *Memorability* refers to how easily users can return to the system after a period of inactivity and recall important functions, features, and interactions.
- *Error resistance and remediation* refers to how well a system prevents errors or handles errors when they occur.
- *Satisfaction* refers to how pleasant the system is to use. Users desire products that are not merely functional, and systems that cause individuals to be miserable are less usable.[10,11]

Two approaches to improving medical device HF are described in the following sections. The first is a design philosophy called human-centered design. The second is a set of design principles, derived from research in cognitive and biological sciences, such as perception, attention, memory, learning, and emotion. These approaches should be used in tandem.

USER-CENTERED DESIGN

The International Organization for Standardization states that user-centered design involves the active involvement of users, clear understanding of user and task requirements, correct allocation of functions between users and technologies, iterative design solutions, and multidisciplinary design.[12] Gould and Lewis[13] articulated 3 tenets for user-centered design:

- An early and constant focus on the users and their tasks.
- Reliance on human-system performance and behavioral data to guide design decisions. Commonly, these data are generated by usability tests, which collect measures such as success and failure rate, error rate, timing, self-report, and user perceptions to reveal problems and barriers.
- Iteration. Good design entails many rounds of design and testing until success rates, error rates, and other outcomes are brought to acceptable levels.

Some common user-centered research methods are described as follows. Some, such as contextual inquiry[14] and ethnography,[15] are aimed at gathering and analyzing user requirements. Broadly, contextual inquiry and ethnography refer to observing and interviewing research participants in their natural place of work (eg, surgical suite, examination room).

Some usability problems can be discovered via systematic inspection of user interfaces and functions without the assistance of authentic end-users (ie, similar to how programmers review and inspect code). These can be implemented quicker and less expensively than full usability tests, and yet enable designers to identify many design flaws early in development. Inspection methods are considered an informal usability evaluation method, because they rely on heuristics and the knowledge of the evaluators. In contrast, empirical techniques assess usability by testing an interface with real users.

One popular usability inspection method is *heuristic evaluation*.[8,16] In heuristic evaluation, 1 or more members of the development team evaluate a product against a list of design principles or rules of thumb. Examples of heuristics, which are particularly useful for medical devices, are provided by Zhang and colleagues,[17] and Graham and colleagues.[18] Evaluations from all reviewers can be aggregated to identify the most common problems and discuss ways to mitigate them. This method has become popular in usability evaluation due to its low cost, low time commitment, and ease of application.

Cognitive walkthrough[19,20] is a method for inspecting the learnability and usability of a system via naturalistic exploration. Developers take on the role of typical users to complete tasks within the system. During the walkthrough, individuals or groups of reviewers reflect on the actions required to complete the tasks and any barriers or confusion encountered. Reviewers might ask questions such as "what would the user be doing at this point?" and "what features in the interface are available to do this?" Importantly, a functional version of the system is not necessary; cognitive walkthroughs can be performed using detailed description of the interface, a mockup, or a working prototype, along with a task scenario or prespecified sequence of actions.[7,21]

Usability testing,[9,22,23] derived from applied experimental psychology, identifies insights about how people use a product or prototype. These expose usability deficiencies, which in turn improve system design. A usability test consists of a series of tasks conducted by authentic end-users or participants who are similar to the target user.[24] Researchers record and analyze objective performance data such as success and failure rate, error frequency, deviation from ideal task path, and task completion time. Additionally, several self-report measures of perceived usability have been developed and used widely.[25]

Usability testing can be used for a variety of purposes depending on the current design stage, including exploration, assessment, comparison, and validation.

- *Exploratory testing* occurs during initial stages of development to evaluate the promise of preliminary concepts. In general, an exploratory test focuses on high-level aspects of the information architecture rather than on fine detail.[9]
- *Formative tests* are conducted early or midway through the development process, usually after high-level design decisions have been made. Formative tests seek to identify and fix usability issues at a detailed level. Tests at this stage typically rely on mockups, prototypes, and tasks that more closely match final products (ie, higher fidelity).
- Comparative tests. When multiple or competing versions are available, *comparison tests* evaluate one design against another. Comparisons can happen at any point in the product development cycle.
- Validation tests. Finally, *validation testing* is usually conducted late in the product development cycle to confirm that features and systems meet predefined standards and benchmarks.

When designing, it is helpful to consider the ways people process information, so that we can present the information and tasks in the most appropriate way. The following sections describe important stages of human information processing, and corresponding design principles and guidelines. For more information on principles and guidelines, see Lee and colleagues,[6] Nielsen,[8] Shneiderman and colleagues,[26] and Zhang and colleagues.[17]

DESIGN PRINCIPLES
Perception

Perception refers to the ability to see, hear, become aware of, and recognize stimuli in our surroundings.[27] Perception relies on more than just sensory organs, such as eyes and ears (bottom-up processing), but it also relies on stored knowledge, experiences, memories, and expectancies (top-down processing). Perception then involves reconciling what our senses tell us with what our brain knows and expects. We can facilitate bottom-up processing in various ways. For example, we can make controls, displays, labels, and text legible from the distance of use. This means that the text must be large enough and provide adequate contrast. Contrast enables us to discriminate between the figure and the background, and is maximized with black text on a white background, although often aesthetics requires another configuration. Use light backgrounds for main areas of displays. Good examples include off whites and grays.[28] It is important that text can be read quickly and easily. Also, for improved perception, not all text is created equal. The perception of text is improved, and the device made more usable, when a familiar and unadorned font is used, when mixed case (rather than all capitals) text is used, and when sans-serif fonts are used on computerized displays and serif fonts are used for hard copy, such as instructions for use.[6,29,30] Finally, include labels on your icons. This reduces ambiguity and speeds recognition.[31]

Sensible grouping of display items and controls facilitates top-down perception. For example, it is advisable to place similar, related, and items used to complete the same task in sequence, close together.[32] Usually white space is helpful to separate display items between groups, but you could also use boxes, borders, color coding, or shape coding. One key is to adhere to user expectancies. Based on experience, people often expect to find items in certain places on a device or screen. It is important to match those expectancies as closely as possible.

Because perception is about recognizing components and groups on a device, we must try to make items as easy to recognize as possible. There are a few ways to do this. One is called pictorial realism.[33] Specifically, it means that a display, icon, or sign should look like the thing it represents. An example of pictorial realism is a print icon that looks like a printer. It is easier to recognize because it looks like the concept it represents. Another tip is to use redundancy gain,[34] which refers to expressing the same information in more than one way. An example is a stop sign, which is red in color, hexagonal in shape, and says STOP. Three cues combine to make the sign more recognizable than any one cue alone.

Finally, perception refers to more than just vision. It is important that auditory alarms, messages, and warnings can be heard in ambient conditions of use.[35] This is difficult these days when so many devices have their own auditory warnings. It should be mentioned that auditory warnings have many qualities, which can be manipulated to make them discriminable. These include volume, frequency, tempo, envelope (for example rising sound or falling sound), and others.[35] This is particularly relevant to the ICU, where health care providers are exposed to numerous technologies all at once,[21] and in which the sheer number of false alarms often causes alarm fatigue.[36] The key is to treat auditory displays such as these with the same attention provided to visual displays.

Attention

The fact that we use the phrase "pay attention" suggests that attention is limited and valuable. Despite our best efforts, we have only so much attention to go around, so we allocate it in ways that help us achieve our goals. You can think of attention as a spotlight. It can be wide and diffuse, shedding a little light on a lot of things, or it can be focused, shedding lots of light on just a few things,[37] but it cannot be both at once. Here are some ways to help users to pay attention to the right things to complete their tasks.

The first approach is to design for minimalism. In 1939, well before many health care technologies, Antoine de Saint-Exupery[38,39] wrote, "a designer has reached perfection not when there is nothing left to add, but when there is nothing left to take away."[a] This captures the essence of minimalist design, encouraging us to avoid clutter, placing only necessary information on the display, because everything else is distracting. Further, color should be used sparingly and consistently. In fact, many designers suggest no more than 4 colors per screen on visual displays,[6,40] and very few colors in icons. The issue is that icons are so small that it is hard to discriminate where one color ends and another begins. This gives it a fuzzy look that makes it hard to recognize.

The best way to get people to pay attention to an item that you want them to notice is through conspicuity[41]; that is, items tend to pop out and capture attention when they differ from their surroundings. These differences can include different shapes, colors, and brightness. On the most rare occasion, for example, an emergency situation, blinking or movement on the display attracts attention strongly. Because it is so distracting though, it should be used only in the most serious situations.

Learning

In a perfect world, all devices would enable us to simply walk up and use them. In this world though, devices often need to be learned. Because humans manage complexity by placing things in categories and hierarchies, learning is facilitated by organization.[42] For example, good graphical user interfaces place items that are related to

---

[a] Actually he wrote "In anything at all, perfection is finally attained not when there is no longer anything to add, but when there is no longer anything to take away." The design profession appropriated and modified the quote slightly.

each other, either because they are similar or are used together in the completion of a task, in close proximity. This enables the user to look at the layout of items and learn the underlying model of the device. Additionally, people spontaneously search for similarities between new situations and previously encountered situations. For this reason, learning is facilitated by analogy and metaphor.[43–45] Indeed, one of the reasons for the success of Apple's Macintosh user interface was because it used the familiar metaphor as a desktop, with files, file folders, and other objects people were already familiar with from the office environment.[46]

Devices are easier to learn when they are consistent, using consistent labeling, placement of information, and color coding.[47] They are also easier to learn if they behave similar to other medical devices used in the same environment and for related tasks. Further, devices are made easier to use when the user is provided with informative feedback, enabling them to understand the device's status at all times.

Generally, people are not motivated to learn how to use a new device; instead, they are motivated to actually use it. Consequently, training and tutorials are most effective if they take place in the context of real work and real tasks. This is one of the benefits of simulation training,[48] designed to re-create the context of use. Each realistic component of the simulation serves as a memory recall aid for during a subsequent actual event. Further, tutorials and documentation should be situated and available during the conduct of these real-world tasks, and easy to find, searchable, and should avoid jargon.

Memory

Peoples' memories are far from perfect.[49] People tend to forget information when they conduct complex tasks, especially if they are distracted or stressed, as they often are in the ICU. Additionally, they tend to forget when trying to integrate information between screens, or even when trying to integrate information from far away on the same screen. It is helpful to provide placeholders for sequential tasks to indicate what step users are on. Also, allow side-by-side comparisons, and do not require users to remember information between screens.

Peoples' ability to recognize information is better than their ability to recall it.[50] So, it is important to avoid command-based systems, which rely on people recalling command names and syntax. Instead provide see-and-point rather than remember-and-type. Provide lists of choices and enable the user to pick from the list.

Language and Communication

Although there are important differences, using a device is similar to communicating with another person. You need to make your intentions known, ask the device to do something for you, interpret what the device did, and then see if it has helped you get closer to your goal. There are some ways to make this communication easier and more satisfying. One way is to use simple and natural dialogue, eliminating extraneous words and graphics as well as unfamiliar or technical terms.[17] Provide text that can be read quickly. This, of course, is related to the notion of minimalism described previously. Another is to use words rather than abbreviations, because abbreviations can be confusing. Finally, be brief and concise, use short words and sentences, and use active voice.

A special type of communication and feedback involves error messages. Error messages are designed to help the user diagnose and recover from problems, informing them of potential failures. It is best to help the user avoid errors to begin with by providing obvious ways to undo, cancel, and redo actions, as well as by providing clearly marked exits. However, when it is necessary to use error messages, they should have the following characteristics[6]:

- Be polite, avoid negative wording, and never blame the users. Avoid intimidating language such as "Catastrophic Failure," or "A Fatal Exception Occurred," or "The Application Will Be Terminated."
- Design the error message for simple step-by step reading (eg, first do this then do that). Put most important information at the beginning of the message. All information should appear in a natural and logical order. Error messages should have 4 components:
  - Describe the problem
  - Describe why it happened
  - Describe a solution
  - Provide access to help and more information

Emotion and Motivation

Typically, when using a medical device, users are trying to be as efficient as possible. They want to feel confident that they are progressing toward their goals of taking care of their patient. To this end, it is important to anticipate the users' needs, providing the information they need, when they need it, and in a helpful format. It is important to simplify task sequences, organizing tasks so that information is easy to find and use. Designers should organize information and functionality by importance of use, frequency of use, and relatedness of meaning. Specifically, important and frequent functions and information should be placed closest to the user. Information and functions that are related to each other, or are used in completion of the same task, should be arranged in close proximity. Finally, choose appropriate defaults,[6] making sure that default values are the ones expected by the user, and do not increase the likelihood of losing data.

It is important, also, to make the user feel in control. Provide a clear beginning and end (closure) for each task. Provide shortcuts for experienced users and frequent operation. These can include function keys, hot keys, command keys, aliases, templates, type-ahead, bookmarks, hot links, history, default values, and so on. Avoid surprising actions, unexpected outcomes, and tedious sequences of actions. Provide informative feedback. Limit interruptions and distractions.

INFORMATION PROCESSING STAGES, DESIGN PRINCIPLES, AND GUIDELINES

Cognitive psychology's information processing stages provide a convenient structure for organizing various design principles and heuristics identified by previous investigators.[6,8,17,26] The principles and guidelines in **Table 1** are ones that the author has found particularly useful in application to medical device design. Most of the principles and guidelines come from Lee and colleagues[6] and Zhang and colleagues.[17] **Table 1** places them into the proper cognitive psychology information processing stages.

DISCUSSION

This article introduced HF considerations in the design of medical devices. Because HF entails designing technology to match human abilities and limitations, and because humans are so complex, it is impossible to cover everything designers need to know in this short introduction. Instead, introducing HF, describing HF methods, discussing cognitive psychology's information processing stages and their implications for

Table 1
Human factors principles and guidelines for medical devices

Category	Principle	Guideline
Perception	Visibility	Make items legible from the distance of use.
		Design text of adequate size and contrast.
		Use light (eg, off whites and very light gray) for the backgrounds for main areas of displays.
	Legibility	Ensure that text can be read quickly and easily.
		Use familiar and unadorned font.
		Use mixed case (rather than all capitals) text.
		Use sans-serif fonts on computerized displays and serif fonts for hard copy.
		Include labels on icons.
	Make items easy to recognize	Pictorial realism: make displays, icons, or signs look like the thing they represent.
		Use redundancy gain: express the same information in more than one way.
	Grouping	Place similar, related, and items used to complete the same task close together.
		Use white space, boxes, borders, color coding, or shape coding to distinguish groups.
		Match user expectancies of item grouping and placement.
	Design good auditory displays	Design auditory alarms and messages to be heard in ambient conditions of use.
		Use all components of sound design, such as volume, frequency, tempo, envelope, and others to make auditory displays discriminable.
Attention	Minimalism	Avoid clutter.
		Use color sparingly.
	Conspicuity	Use uniqueness of color, shape, and so forth to make critical items stand out from the background.
		For emergencies, use blinking or motion to attract attention.
Learning	Organization	Organize controls and displays in sensible categories and hierarchies.
		Make use of analogies and design metaphors.
	Consistency	Be consistent in labeling, placement of information, color coding.
		Use appropriate and expected defaults.
		When possible, be consistent with other medical devices used in the same environment and for related tasks.
	Feedback	Provide informative feedback.
		Ensure user is informed about the device's status at all times.
	Training and tutorials	Situate training and tutorials in the context of real work and real tasks.
		Make training and tutorials easy to find, searchable, and without jargon.
Memory	Placeholders	Provide placeholders for sequential tasks to indicate what step you are on.
	Side-by-side comparisons	Allow side-by-side comparisons, and do not require users to remember information between screens.
	Use recognition over recall	Avoid command-based systems, which rely on recalling command names and syntax.
		Provide see-and-point rather than remember-and-type.
		Provide lists of choices and enable the user to pick from the list.

(continued on next page)

Table 1 (continued)		
Category	**Principle**	**Guideline**
Language and communication	Use simple and natural dialogue	Avoid unfamiliar or technical terms.
		Eliminate extraneous words and graphics.
		Provide text that can be read quickly.
		Use words rather than abbreviations.
		Be brief and concise. Use short words and sentences, and use active voice.
	Keep users informed	Inform users of progress toward task completion.
		Make error messages polite.
		Never blame the user.
		Avoid intimidating language.
		Design error messages for simple step-by-step reading (eg, first do this then do that).
		Put most important information at the beginning of messages.
		Write error messages with 4 components: (1) describe the problem; (2) describe why it happened; (3) describe a solution; and (4) provide access to help and more information.
Emotion and motivation	Confidence	Help users feel confident that they are progressing toward their goal.
		Attempt to anticipate the users' needs by providing the information they need, when they need it, and in a helpful format.
	Simplify task sequences	Organize tasks so that information is easy to find and use.
		Choose appropriate and expected defaults.
		Organize information and functionality by importance of use, frequency of use, and relatedness of meaning.
	Provide feeling of control	Make the user feel in control.
		Avoid surprising actions, unexpected outcomes.
		Avoid tedious sequences of actions.
		Provide informative feedback.
		Limit interruptions and distractions.
		Provide a clear beginning and end (closure) for each task.
		Provide shortcuts for experienced users and frequent operation.

design, and finally providing a table of design principles and guidelines will need to suffice.

Key to understanding HF is the insight that the most complex component of your medical device, and key to its success and safety, is the user attempting to operate it. This human component requires just as much attention (in fact probably more) than the mechanical, electrical, or other considerations. This requires early and constant focus on the user, evidence-based design decisions, and fast iteration.[13] In short, it requires user-centered design.

REFERENCES

1. Angus DC, Kelley MA, Schmitz RJ. Current and projected workforce requirements for care. JAMA 2000;284(21):2762–70.

2. Halpern NA, Bettes L, Greenstein R. Federal and nationwide intensive care units and healthcare costs: 1986-1992. Crit Care Med 1994;22(12):2001–7.

3. Carayon P, Gürses AP. A human factors engineering conceptual framework of nursing workload and patient safety in intensive care units. Intensive Crit Care Nurs 2005;21(5):284–301.
4. Donchin Y, Gopher D, Olin M, et al. A look into the nature and causes of human errors in the intensive care unit. Crit Care Med 1995;23(2):294–300.
5. Garrouste-Orgeas M, Philippart F, Bruel C, et al. Overview of medical errors and adverse events. Ann Intensive Care 2012;2(1):1–9.
6. Lee JD, Wickens CD, Liu Y, et al. Designing for people: an introduction to human factors engineering. 3rd edition. Charleston (SC): CreateSpace; 2017.
7. Roscoe RD, Craig NJ, Branaghan RJ, et al. Human systems engineering and educational technology. In: Roscoe RD, Craig SD, Douglas I, editors. End-user considerations in educational technology design. IGI Global; 2017. p. 1–30.
8. Nielsen J. Usability engineering. Cambridge (MA): Academic Press; 1993.
9. Rubin J, Chisnell D. Handbook of usability testing: how to plan, design and conduct effective tests. Indianapolis (IN): Wiley Publishing; 2008.
10. Norman DA. Emotional design: why we love (or hate) everything things. Philadelphia: Basic Books; 2005.
11. Norman DA. The design of everyday things: revised and expanded edition. Philadelphia: Basic Books; 2013.
12. Jokela T, Iivari N, Matero J, et al. The standard of user-centered design and the standard definition of usability: analyzing ISO 13407 against ISO 9241-11. Proceedings of the Latin American conference on human-computer interaction. New York: ACM; 2003. p. 53–60.
13. Gould JD, Lewis C. Designing for usability: key principles and what designers think. Commun ACM 1985;28(3):300–11.
14. Holtzblatt K, Beyer H. Contextual design: design for life. New York: Morgan Kaufmann; 2016.
15. Hammersley M, Atkinson P. Ethnography: principles in practice. 3rd edition. London: Routledge; 2007.
16. Nielsen J, Budiu R. Mobile usability. San Francisco (CA): New Riders Press; 2013.
17. Zhang J, Johnson TR, Patel VL, et al. Using usability heuristics to evaluate patient safety of medical devices. J Biomed Inform 2003;36(1):23–30.
18. Graham MJ, Kubose TK, Jordan D, et al. Heuristic evaluation of infusion pumps: implications for patient safety in intensive care units. Int J Med Inform 2004; 73(11):771–9.
19. Polson PG, Lewis C, Rieman J, et al. Cognitive walkthroughs: a method for theory-based evaluation of user interfaces. Int J Man Mach Stud 1992;36(5):741–73.
20. Sears A, Hess DJ. Cognitive walkthroughs: understanding the effect of task-description detail on evaluator performance. Int J Hum Comput Interact 1999; 11(3):185–200.
21. Bhutkar G, Katre D, Ray G, et al. Usability Model for Medical User Interface of Ventilator System in Intensive Care Unit. In: Campos P, Clemmensen T, Nocera JA, et al, editors. Work Analysis and HCI. 3rd Human Work Interaction Design (HWID). Copenhagen (Denmark): Springer; 2012. p. 46–64. Available at: https://hal.inria.fr/hal-01463377/document.
22. Dumas JS, Redish J. A practical guide to usability testing. Portland (OR): Intellect Books; 1999.
23. Kortum P. Usability assessment: how to measure the usability of products, services, and systems. Santa Monica (CA): Human, Factors, and Ergonomics Society; 2016.
24. Wichansky AM. Usability testing in 2000 and beyond. Ergonomics 2000;43(7): 998–1006.

25. Tullis TS, Albert W. Measuring the user experience: collecting, analyzing, and presenting usability metrics. New York: Morgan Kaufman; 2013.
26. Shneiderman B, Plaisant C, Cohen MS, et al. Designing the user interface: strategies for effective human-computer interaction. Upper Saddle River (NJ): Pearson; 2016.
27. Goldstein EB, Brockmole J. Sensation and perception. Boston (MA): Cengage Learning; 2016.
28. Lavie T, Tractinsky N. Assessing dimensions of perceived visual aesthetics of web sites. Int J Hum Comput Stud 2004;60(3):269–98.
29. Bernard ML, Chaparro BS, Mills MM, et al. Comparing the effects of text size and format on the readability of computer-displayed Times New Roman and Arial text. Int J Hum Comput Stud 2003;59(6):823–35.
30. Legge GE, Bigelow CA. Does print size matter for reading. A review of findings from vision science and typography. J Vis 2011;11(5):8, 1-22.
31. Wiedenbeck S. The use of icons and labels in an end user application program: an empirical study of learning and retention. Behav Inf Technol 1999; 18(2):68–82.
32. Branaghan RJ, Covas-Smith CM, Jackson KD, et al. Using knowledge structures to redesign an instructor–operator station. Appl Ergon 2011;42(6):934–40.
33. Wickens CD. Aviation Displays. In: Tsang PS, Vidulich MA, editors. Principles and Practice of Aviation Psychology. Mahwah (NJ): Lawrence Erlbaum Associates; 2003. p. 147–99.
34. Egeth HE, Mordkoff JT. Redundancy gain revisited: Evidence for parallel processing of separable dimensions. In: Lockhead GR, Pomerantz JR, editors. The perception of structure: Essays in honor of Wendell R. Garner. Washington, DC: American Psychological Association; 1991. p. 131–43.
35. Stanton NA, Edworthy J. Human factors in auditory warnings. Brookfield (VT): Ashgate; 1999.
36. Graham KC, Cvach M. Monitor alarm fatigue: standardizing use of physiological monitors and decreasing nuisance alarms. Am J Crit Care 2010;19(1):28–34.
37. Treisman AM, Gelade G. A feature-integration theory of attention. Cogn Psychol 1980;12(1):97–136.
38. de St. Exupery A. Wind sand and stars. New York: Harcourt Inc; 1967. Trans. Lewis Galantiere.
39. Donahue GM. Usability and the bottom line. IEEE Softw 2001;18(1):31–7.
40. Horton WK. The icon book: visual symbols for computer systems and documentation. New York: John Wiley & Sons, Inc; 1994.
41. Engel FL. Visual conspicuity, visual search and fixation tendencies of the eye. Vis Res 1977;17(1):95–108.
42. Kieras DE, Bovair S. The role of a mental model in learning to operate a device. Cogn Sci 1984;8(3):255–73.
43. Carroll JM, Mack RL. Metaphor, computing systems, and active learning. Int J Man Mach Stud 1985;22(1):39–57.
44. Cvach M. Monitor alarm fatigue: an integrative review. Biomed Instrum Technol 2012;46(4):268–77.
45. Duit R. On the role of analogies and metaphors in learning science. Sci Educ 1991;75(6):649–72.
46. Moran T, Zhai S. Beyond the desktop metaphor in seven dimensions. In: Kaptelinin V, Czerwinski M, editors. Beyond the desktop metaphor: designing integrated digital work environments, vol. 1. The MIT Press; 2007. p. 335–55.

47. Nielsen J. Coordinating user interfaces for consistency. ACM SIGCHI Bulletin 1989;20(3):63–5.
48. Ziv A, Wolpe PR, Small SD, et al. Simulation-based medical education: an ethical imperative. Acad Med 2003;78(8):783–8.
49. Baddeley AD. Human memory: theory and practice. New York: Psychology Press; 1997.
50. Gillund G, Shiffrin RM. A retrieval model for both recognition and recall. Psychol Rev 1984;91(1):1.

Informatics Solutions for Application of Decision-Making Skills

Christine W. Nibbelink, PhD, RN[a],*, Janay R. Young, DNP, RN[b],
Jane M. Carrington, PhD, RN[c], Barbara B. Brewer, PhD, RN, MALS, MBA[c]

KEYWORDS

- Nursing informatics • Electronic health record • Clinical data • Clinical databases
- Clinical decision support systems • Nursing practice • Critical care nursing

KEY POINTS

- Decision-making in critical care nursing practice is highly demanding and is essential to quality patient outcomes.
- Nursing practice in critical care environments involves caring for patients with complex disease processes and requires in-depth, evidence-based understanding of pathophysiology and treatments to provide effective patient care.
- Informatics tools provide important support for nurse decision-making through integration of patient information with evidence.

INTRODUCTION

Poor decision-making has been linked with up to 98,000 deaths in hospitals each year.[1] Research indicates that critical care nurses make 238 decisions per hour.[2] Nursing informatics solutions represent one important effort to improve patient outcomes and support nursing practice. Nursing informatics is a field of science that combines the sciences of nursing, information, computers, and cognition to provide better access to patient information and support nursing practice.[3] The goal of nursing informatics is to facilitate progression of patient data to information and

Conflicts of Interest and Source of Funding: The authors declare that they have no conflicts of interest associated with this article. This publication was supported by the National Library of Medicine of the National Institutes of Health under Award Number T15LM011271. The content is solely the responsibility of the authors and does not necessarily represent the official views of the National Institutes of Health.
[a] Department of Biomedical Informatics, University of California, San Diego, 9500 Gilman Drive, La Jolla, CA 92093, USA; [b] Special Immunology Associates, El Rio Community Health Center, 1701 West Saint Mary's Road # 160, Tucson, AZ 85745, USA; [c] University of Arizona, College of Nursing, 1305 North Martin, Tucson, AZ 85721, USA
* Corresponding author. 9500 Gilman Drive, La Jolla, CA 92093.
E-mail address: cnibbelink@ucsd.edu

wisdom to improve the patient condition.[3] Nursing informatics currently includes many tools aimed at facilitation of these efforts. The purpose of this article was to discuss the utilization of electronic health record (EHR), clinical data, and Clinical Decision Support System (CDSS) tools to support decision-making in critical care nursing practice.

BACKGROUND

Critical care nurses coordinate care for patients with highly complex and potentially unstable illnesses.[4] This requires critical care nurses to work within health care teams to maintain awareness of a patient's current status to limit and respond to complications with an end goal of improved patient outcomes.[4] This high level of nursing care requires specialized education, knowledge, and skills for effective response to changes in patient status.[4] Despite experience and training of nurses caring for complex patients, memory and rapid data processing can interfere with timely and correct decision-making. The EHR can assist in decision-making. In part due to Meaningful Use promoted by Health Information Technology for Economic and Clinical Health (HITECH) Acts as part of the American Recovery and Reinvestment Act of 2009, CDSS is required to facilitate effective use of the EHR in health care to improve patient outcomes.[5]

INFORMATICS TOOLS IN CRITICAL CARE
Electronic Health Record

The EHR serves as the core technology within the health care setting. The EHR functions to collect, store, and make available important patient information to support decision-making and care planning. Nurses manage thousands of data points each shift, reflective of the complex nature of critically ill patients.[5] This is successful in part due to 2 characteristics of the EHR. First, embedded within the EHR are other technologies, such as CDSS, algorithms as alerts and early warning systems, and interfaces connecting, for example, infusion pump, hospital bed, and hemodynamic monitor data. Data from these devices have the potential of triggering an early warning alert (a problem is likely) or CDSS an actual problem (critical value). Second, the EHR supports data entry of patient information, which is a critical element for other embedded applications, such as acuity scale, pressure ulcer risk scale, and pain scale.[6]

Despite these characteristics of the EHR, effectiveness of the EHR as a technology to guide clinical decision-making is inconclusive. The current EHR is effective as a data entry system, it falls short with data retrieval threatening decision-making.[6] Despite this, the federal mandate, Meaningful Use, sought to increase effective use of the EHR for improved patient outcomes.[7] This mandate sought to attach reimbursement to effective use of the EHR that includes use of embedded technologies to enhance decision-making.[8] Meaningful Use guidelines seek to enhance accessibility of information in the EHR for better patient outcomes.[7] Unfortunately, nursing research finds that although the EHR is effective as a data entry tool, data retrieval is limited.[6]

Clinical Databases

Clinical databases are a collection of clinical data that exist "behind" the front-facing screens of the EHR and allow for data to be captured from basic and advanced hemodynamic monitoring devices and then integrated with the EHR. Monitoring devices used in the intensive care unit (ICU), such as arterial pressure or pulmonary artery catheters, capture semicontinuous values that allow for nurse-driven monitoring and evaluation of the therapeutic effect of interventions.[9] The monitoring devices communicate with the EHR over a secure network, wirelessly or directly with an Ethernet converter.[10] The ICU nurse determines the frequency with which the data are captured, validates that the data collected are accurate, and then saves them to the patient's permanent EHR. Examples of patient data that can be mined for use in decision support are broad. Patients requiring ICU care may experience circulatory failure requiring immediate nursing assessment of basic and advanced hemodynamics for minute-to-minute assessment. These data could be combined with evidence for best practice. Clinical data that are directly from the EHR inform specific CDSSs.

There are some larger health care systems in which patient data from the EHR are populated and stored in databases stored in a clinical data warehouse, which is used for data analysis and reporting.[11] Clinical data enter the warehouse in a de-identified state. An interested clinician or scientist can obtain clinical data sets (based on specific International Classification of Diseases, Ninth or 10th Revision codes, demographic information, and so forth) and then process, transform, mine, and evaluate the data to answer clinical or research questions.[11] The data in the clinical data warehouse are used primarily for research at this time point; however, these data hold great potential for using statistical techniques to model patients who share characteristics toward the development of more informed CDSSs that are data driven to deliver specific nurse care.

The clinical data stored in clinical data warehouse can be analyzed and studied to identify patterns and relationships in a method called data mining.[11,12] Data mining is the process of extracting data from large datasets to determine relationships and patterns that can be used for formulating predictive models.[12] The knowledge generated from data mining can inform and enhance the decision-making process and to develop the CDSS, which could eventually be used for immediate clinical feedback.[11] Nursing practice includes determination of appropriate pharmacologic and nonpharmacologic interventions.[9] Nursing decision support could provide recommendations that include assessment of mixed venous oxygen saturation (SvO2), through repeated blood withdrawal from the pulmonary artery catheter, as an indicator of the oxygen supply/demand balance.[13] SvO2 less than 50% requires the ICU nurse to perform a rapid patient assessment and to provide physiologic optimization, which may include oxygen administration, fluid infusion, diuretics, vasopressors, and/or inotropes.[13] Through the integration of evidence with clinical data, nurse decision-making may be more effectively supported. For example, clinical data including measurement of fluid intake and output, daily weight, vital signs, and SVO2, can be used to develop a CDSS to titrate diuretics to improve diuresis.

Clinical Decision Support Systems

CDSSs are computer software tools designed to facilitate decision-making through connecting evidence with patient status.[14] Use of CDSSs can improve guideline compliance through warnings, alerts, and advice.[14,15] The CDSS is an increasingly important tool in nursing practice. Research identifies the CDSS as supporting decision-making in time-limited circumstances leading to improved patient outcomes. Nursing research is inconclusive in demonstrating effectiveness of CDSSs in nursing practice[16]; however, Meaningful Use requirements and the demanding nature of decision-making in nursing practice, require that the CDSS will continue to be developed as an important part of nursing practice. Barriers to CDSS use must be better understood and addressed. Examples of CDSS tools, factors associated with nurse use of CDSS, suggestions for CDSS improvement, and CDSS and nursing care of ICU patients are addressed.

Clinical Decision Support System tools

No all-inclusive list of the CDSS exists.[17,18] Many tools that support decision-making may not be commonly thought of as CDSSs.[17,18] Many examples of CDSSs exist, including paper decision support tools, order sets, parameters for patient care, patient data, and patient monitors.[16-18] Nursing literature does describe examples of tools that are more commonly thought of as CDSS. Examples of CDSS tools identified in the literature include information management, focusing attention, and patient-specific consultation.[19] Information management CDSS includes patient education material, info buttons, or guidelines for practice.[19] Another type of CDSS focuses the attention of nurses. Examples of focusing attention include drug-to-drug interaction warnings and fall risk warnings.[19] The final type of CDSS is patient-specific consultation. Ideal patient-specific consultation CDSS provides the health care professional with a broad array of patient information combined with guidelines to support decision-making.[19] Thus, effective and comprehensive nurse documentation in the EHR is essential for patient-specific decision support. Elements such as depression scoring, patient goals, and body mass index provide information that could enhance patient-specific decision support.[19]

Factors associated with Clinical Decision Support System use

Nurses' interaction with CDSS as a decision support tool is influenced by a variety of factors. Some research indicates nurses describe CDSS as supportive of decision-making.[14] Inexperienced nurses do find CDSS supportive of their decisions.[20] However, more experienced nurses use CDSS less frequently than inexperienced nurses.[20-22]

Many barriers to nurse use of the CDSS in practice exist, including problems with usability and support of nursing knowledge.[14] In addition, nurses may ignore evidence-based recommendations made by the CDSS, indicating a failure in the design of the system.[23,24] Nurses also may bypass recommendations provided by the CDSS if they believe that their own or a colleague's advice is more appropriate for the patient care situation.[14,16] An impediment to nurse interaction with the CDSS could be associated with a lack of trust in CDSS effectiveness.[15,25] Nurses must believe that the CDSS will support their practice to regard it as an important device that provides evidence with which to base decision-making. Excessive alerts also diminish nurses' willingness to interact with the CDSS when decision-making.[15,26] Frequent alerts, rather than keeping the nurse focused on evidence-based guidelines, create a negative use experience for nurses leading to decreased interaction with this tool. Although the CDSS does provide support for nurse decision-making in some circumstances (such as reminders to check heart rate when administering beta blockers), many areas for advancement need to be addressed.

Improvement of the Clinical Decision Support System

Several suggestions for CDSS improvement are described in nursing literature. To begin with, the design of the CDSS must be user focused for enhanced usability for the nurse end user.[25,27,28] User focus would include CDSS design and identification of the end users' physical, perceptual, and cognitive needs.[25,29] Timing of CDSS information is essential. Research identifies that nurse use of the CDSS increased when the CDSS information fit with nursing workflow.[16] The CDSS must fit the nurse user role. For example, charge nurse workflow and bedside nurse workflow present different CDSS user needs.[30] Excessive alerts sent to nurses using the CDSS lead to ignored messages.[31] CDSS tools that do not meet end user needs lead to reduced access to evidence for decision-making.

To better support acute care nurse decision-making, the end user should participate in design. One study designed a nurse role–specific CDSS with characteristics identified by the participating acute care nurses as important for CDSS.[30] Nurses described the predominant needs of CDSS for acute care nursing practice: provide a picture of the patient's status over the course of time, support nurse autonomy, and align with the individual needs of the patient.[30] Through inclusion of the end user in the development of the CDSS, specific decision support needs can be addressed, potentially resulting in a more effectively implemented CDSS in acute care.

Use of the Clinical Decision Support System in acute care nursing practice

Effective CDSS could support decision-making with many patient populations. A logic model exists in the background of the EHR system, connecting evidence-based practice to the CDSS alert and recommendations. The highly complex nature of ICU nursing care requires excellent decision-making skills in conjunction with the data that exist in the EHR and experience of the clinician. The CDSS with evidence-based logic guides nurses toward effective decision-making in anticipation of medication side effects. Evidence-based clinical decision support tools are also effective toward determining the best diagnostic tests. CDSSs could be constructed to include alerts to test for laboratory studies specific to patient diagnoses.[32]

It is important to point out that at this time point, CDSSs are patient specific, such as with recommendations to check vital signs when administering a particular medication, and are not designed for a specific diagnosis. For example, a message from the CDSS could read "Patient heart rate less than 50 and consider hold Digitalis is due" or "Patient's K is <3.5 and patient on diuretic consider potassium supplement." Rather, designers, nursing informatics scientists, and those in advance practice, work together using best evidence to analyze connections within data. For example, data collection for patients in the ICU can include abnormal values in pressure monitoring, medications, laboratory values, and so forth, that tell a story about the patient and are applied to specific patients with particular diagnosis to provide the nurse with more information on which to base decisions. As we move forward with data-driven care and predictive modeling, CDSSs will provide enhanced information for improved decision support.

Research indicates that improved guideline use in the provision of acute care is needed.[15] Despite this, health care professionals continue to resist use of the CDSS in the care of complex ICU patients, believing that the CDSS may make mistakes and that their own experience is more valuable than CDSS advice.[15] In addition, in a study surveying 36 cardiologists and 126 heart failure specialty nurses on the use of the CDSS in patient care, 70% of study participants stated that they would not miss significant changes, such as assessment or laboratory values, in patient status.[15] Nurses and cardiologists identify that the CDSS adds knowledge to their provision of care, but believe that CDSS advice must always be confirmed by the health care professional.[15] Use of the Internet, number of years using e-mail, and number of years using computers enhanced trust of the CDSS with participants of this study.[15] Alerts, although designed to increase adoption of guidelines in practice, may lead to resistance to CDSS use.[15] Investigators theorized that alerts led users to feel less autonomous in their practice.[15] Understanding how CDSS systems work reduced barriers to use of the CDSS, leading investigators to emphasize the importance of user attitude toward the CDSS for best patient outcomes.[15]

Clearly, the CDSS must be improved to better support nursing practice. Nurse users of the CDSS must be involved in design of the CDSS to ensure that decision support needs will be met. CDSS advice must include patient-specific advice and be provided in accordance with nursing workflow for greater acceptance. Development of the CDSS with recognition of the specific end user needs in terms of nursing role and experience level to guide user focused alerts could increase CDSS acceptance.

Predictive Analytics

Within the umbrella of precision health, predictive analytics has emerged. The concepts of precision medicine and nursing are gaining momentum in our data-rich health care system. Predictive analytics are used to analyze genomic, environment, and life style (precision medicine)[33] and evidence-based and personalized patient care (precision nursing)[34] toward quality outcomes and patient safety.[33,34] Both concepts are evolving as we gain access to and understanding of patient data within the EHR. It is here that we find patterns emerge with patient characteristics and outcomes to inform predictive analytics.

Predictive analytics uses strategies with machine learning or teaching the computer to think and process data. CDSSs developed using this approach are generally referred to as "data driven" and can be applied to several patient conditions, such as sepsis.[35] Using data from the EHR and database and the logic from the CDSS, models can be created that provide "predictions" of patient outcomes based on patient characteristics. And, with these predictions, specify the care the patient requires for a quality outcome.

Imagine nurses admitting a patient into the ICU and once the data are entered in the EHR, algorithms are working in the background to find key characteristics of the patient to determine their precise care needs and predictions of the patient risks for complications or delays in discharge.

Application to Practice

Patients in the ICU are monitored and managed using many devices that collect an enormous amount of data that could, in the near future, be used to develop an algorithm in the background of the EHR and uses predictive models to determine the patient risk for complications. Techniques in computer science, natural language processing, and machine learning teach the computer to mine EHR data to predict patient outcomes or risk for increased morbidity or mortality. Specific to cardiac disease and intensive care, predictive analytics could be applied to predict patient outcomes with acute coronary syndrome and heart failure.[36–39] Furthermore, similar models are being tested to determine acuity from EHR data.[40] These examples, and no doubt many more that have yet to be published, remain in the development and test environment and will surely become embedded within the EHR in the near future. Another key point to these algorithms and clinical impact is that these will improve the decision-making process. Rather than an alert informing the nurse that his or her patient has an abnormal laboratory value or vital sign, these advanced CDSSs can provide a risk estimate of the patient for morbidity or mortality and acuity, providing a higher level of decision support for the nurse. Although this is a developing science, future applications of this technology applied to cardiovascular patients could predict risk and medication surveillance, precision medicine and nursing decision support, and population health.[41]

Applications for big data could include important considerations associated with population health, including quality-of-care factors and phenotyping to more precisely diagnose and treat patients with cardiovascular disease.[41] Although prescriptive analytics that could support medical decision-making for care of patients with cardiovascular disease do not currently exist, the possibilities for future applications is strong.[41]

Therefore, applications designed for nursing practice also could include predictive analytics.

DISCUSSION AND RECOMMENDATIONS

From the information provided previously in this article, we present recommendations for effective use of technology to increase patient safety. Several technologies are used to monitor patient status and assist in decision-making; for example, data from technologies (telemetry monitor, pulse oximetry, to glucometer) provide the EHR with data that could then trigger an alert from the CDSS to assist in decision-making. An abundance of data are collected each shift, and when organized, can be used to learn more about our patients and inform care for populations, beyond the current patient. Based on this, we propose the following recommendations. First, training new staff to use patient-monitoring technology and the EHR should include content that explains nurses' contributions to the data collected and value of the data toward decision-making. Second, unit and organization administration should work together to design information systems that use data within the EHR to increase decision-making support and understanding of patients and populations. Third, build interdisciplinary teams for the purpose of discovering best practice from the clinical data and literature. Finally, exploit big data and databases for information that improves care for the patient, guiding all aspects of patient care and teaching.

Clinical data can be applied to develop predictive models and CDSSs to inform clinical decisions and tailor clinical management of patients with critical illness.[41] Use of predictive models and CDSSs in nursing can allow for individualized therapeutic decisions and guidance of effective use of limited health care resources to improve both quality and efficiency in care, leading to improved patient outcomes.[41] The savings from use of big data in health care are estimated to be in the billions per year in the United States, due to waste reduction and improved outcomes.[42] To date, there are few examples in the literature on predictive and prescriptive analytics to inform medical therapeutic decisions or guide ICU nurses' decisions and interventions.[41,43] Rather, general CDSS alerts are available for general care whereby patients in the ICU still benefit, such as diet, medications, and laboratory assays. With the development of predictive analytics and advances of precision medicine and nursing, CDSSs will become more focused.

SUMMARY

Nursing science is behind medical science in understanding CDSS use in nursing practice.[14] Better understanding of factors associated with nurse use of CDSSs in patient care could facilitate use of CDSSs in nursing practice. In the complex, time-limited care of critically ill patients, decisions must be made based on evidence for best outcomes.[44] The EHR, clinical data, and CDSSs are important informatics tools that can facilitate integration of evidence in nursing practice. Future research that explores experienced nurses' use of CDSSs, facilitation of decision-making in time-limited situations at the appropriate time in the nurses' workflow, and incorporation of nurse user needs in CDSS design could enhance nurse use of CDSSs and lead to better patient outcomes.

REFERENCES

1. Kohn LT, Corrigan JM, Donaldson MS. Errors in health care: a leading cause of death and injury. To err is human: building a safer health system. 1999. Available at: http://www.nap.edu/download.php?record_id=9728#.

2. Bucknall T. Critical care nurses' decision-making activities in the natural clinical setting. J Clin Nurs 2000;9(1):25–35.
3. McGonigle D, Hunter K, Sipes C, et al. Why nurses need to understand nursing informatics. AORN J 2014;100(3):324–7.
4. Lakanmaa R-L, Suominen T, Perttilä J, et al. Competence requirements in intensive and critical care nursing–still in need of definition? A Delphi study. Intensive Crit Care Nurs 2012;28(6):329–36.
5. McCormick K. Intensive care unit, emergency room, and operating room. In: Saba V, McCormick K, editors. Essentials of computers for nurses. Philadelphia: Lippincott; 1986. p. 300–29.
6. Carrington JME, Effken JA. Strengths and limitations of the electronic health record for documenting clinical events. Comput Inform Nurs 2011;29(6):360–7.
7. Fife CE, Walker D, Thomson B. Electronic health records, registries, and quality measures: what? why? how? Adv Wound Care (New Rochelle) 2013;2(10): 598–604.
8. Blumenthal D, Tavenner M. The "meaningful use" regulation for electronic health records. N Engl J Med 2010;363(6):501–4.
9. De Backer D. Is there a role for invasive hemodynamic monitoring in acute heart failure management? Curr Heart Fail Rep 2015;12(3):197–204.
10. Zaleski J. Integrating device data into the electronic medical record. Erlangen (Germany): Publicis Publishing; 2008.
11. Chen ES, Sarkar IN. Mining the electronic health record for disease knowledge. Methods Mol Biol 2014;1159:269–86.
12. Zaki M, Meira W. Data mining and analysis: fundamental concepts and algorithms. New York: Cambridge University Press; 2014.
13. Booker KJ. Hemodynamic monitoring in critical care, in critical care nursing: monitoring and treatment for advanced nursing practice. Hoboken (NJ): John Wiley & Sons, Inc; 2015.
14. Anderson JA, Willson P. Clinical decision support systems in nursing: synthesis of the science for evidence-based practice. Comput Inform Nurs 2008;26(3):151–8.
15. de Vries AE, van der Wal MH, Nieuwenhuis MM, et al. Perceived barriers of heart failure nurses and cardiologists in using clinical decision support systems in the treatment of heart failure patients. BMC Med Inform Decis Mak 2013;13:54.
16. Piscotty R, Kalisch B. Nurses' use of clinical decision support: a literature review. Comput Inform Nurs 2014;32(12):562–8.
17. Clinical decision support. How to implement EHRs. 2017. Available at: https://www.healthit.gov/providers-professionals/clinical-decision-support-cds. Accessed June 16, 2017.
18. Clinical decision support: more than just 'alerts' tipsheet. 2014. Available at: https://www.healthit.gov/sites/default/files/clinicaldecisionsupport_tipsheet.pdf. Accessed June 16, 2017.
19. Bakken S, Currie LM, Lee NJ, et al. Integrating evidence into clinical information systems for nursing decision support. Int J Med Inform 2008;77(6):413–20.
20. Dowding D, Randell R, Mitchell N, et al. Experience and nurses use of computerised decision support systems. Stud Health Technol Inform 2009;146:506–10.
21. Harrison RL, Lyerla F. Using nursing clinical decision support systems to achieve meaningful use. Comput Inform Nurs 2012;30(7):380–5.
22. Yuan MJ, Finley GM, Long J, et al. Evaluation of user interface and workflow design of a bedside nursing clinical decision support system. Interact J Med Res 2013;2(1):e4.

23. Lyerla F, LeRouge C, Cooke DA, et al. A nursing clinical decision support system and potential predictors of head-of-bed position for patients receiving mechanical ventilation. Am J Crit Care 2010;19(1):39–47.

24. Boston-Fleischhauer C. Enhancing healthcare process design with human factors engineering and reliability science, part 2: applying the knowledge to clinical documentation systems. J Nurs Adm 2008;38(2):84–9.

25. Boy GA. The handbook of human-machine interaction: a human-centered design approach. Burlington (VT): Ashgate; 2011.

26. Campion TR Jr, May AK, Waitman LR, et al. Characteristics and effects of nurse dosing over-rides on computer-based intensive insulin therapy protocol performance. J Am Med Inform Assoc 2011;18(3):251–8.

27. Effken J, McGonigle D, Mastrian KG. The human-technology interface. In: McGonigle D, Mastrian KG, editors. Nursing informatics and the foundation of knowledge. 3rd edition. Burlington (MA): Ashgate; 2015. p. 201–16.

28. Johnson CM, Johnson TR, Zhang J. A user-centered framework for redesigning health care interfaces. J Biomed Inform 2005;38(1):75–87.

29. Staggers N, Parks PL. Description and initial applications of the Staggers & Parks nurse-computer interaction framework. Comput Nurs 1993;11(6):282–90.

30. Jeffery AD, Novak LL, Kennedy B, et al. Participatory design of probability-based decision support tools for in-hospital nurses. J Am Med Inform Assoc 2017;24(6):1102–10.

31. Campion TR Jr, Waitman LR, Lorenzi NM, et al. Barriers and facilitators to the use of computer-based intensive insulin therapy. Int J Med Inform 2011;80(12):863–71.

32. Paul S, Hice A. Role of the acute care nurse in managing patients with heart failure using evidence-based care. Crit Care Nurs Q 2014;37(4):357–76.

33. National Library of Medicine. What is precision medicine? Your guide to understanding gentoc conditions 2018. Available at: https://ghr.nlm.nih.gov/primer/precisionmedicine/definition. Accessed January 17, 2018.

34. Nursing Knowledge 2016. Paper presented at: Big Data Science Conference. Minneapolis (MN), June 1-3, 2016.

35. Tsoukalas A, Albertson T, Tagkopoulos I. From data to optimal decision making: a data-driven, probabilistic machine learning approach to decision support for patients with sepsis. JMIR Med Inform 2015;3(1):e11.

36. Churpek MM, Yuen TC, Park SY, et al. Using electronic health record data to develop and validate a prediction model for adverse outcomes on the wards. Crit Care Med 2014;42(4):841–8.

37. Escobar GJ, LaGuardia JC, Turk BJ, et al. Early detection of impending physiologic deterioration among patients who are not in intensive care: development of predictive models using data from an automated electronic medical record. J Hosp Med 2012;7(5):388–95.

38. Panahiazar M, Taslimitehrani V, Pereira N, et al. Using EHRs and machine learning for heart failure survival analysis. Stud Health Technol Inform 2015;216:40–4.

39. Sladojević M, Čanković M, Čemerlić S, et al. Data mining approach for in-hospital treatment outcome in patients with acute coronary syndrome. Med Pregl 2015;68(5–6):157–61.

40. Lee J, Maslove DM. Customization of a severity of illness score using local electronic medical record data. J Intensive Care Med 2015;32(1):38–47.

41. Rumsfeld JS, Joynt KE, Maddox TM. Big data analytics to improve cardiovascular care: promise and challenges. Nat Rev Cardiol 2016;13(6):350–9.

42. Raghupathi W, Raghupathi V. Big data analytics in healthcare: promise and potential. Health Inf Sci Syst 2014;2(1):3.
43. Jeffery AD. Methodological challenges in examining the impact of healthcare predictive analytics on nursing-sensitive patient outcomes. Comput Inform Nurs 2015;33(6):258–64.
44. Yancy CW, Jessup M, Bozkurt B, et al. 2013 ACCF/AHA guideline for the management of heart failure: a report of the American College of Cardiology Foundation/American Heart Association Task Force on Practice Guidelines. J Am Coll Cardiol 2013;62(16):e147–239.

Advocating for Greater Usability in Clinical Technologies
The Role of the Practicing Nurse

Karen Dunn Lopez, PhD, MPH, RN[a],*, Linda Fahey, DNP, MSN[b]

KEYWORDS

- Usability • Nursing informatics • Electronic health records • Clinical nursing
- Empower

KEY POINTS

- Intensive care nurses use multiple technologies to perform an array of patient care tasks. For technologies to be useful, they must have utility and be highly usable.
- Electronic health records mediate many of nurses' tasks, and usability problems with these records can have unintended consequences that harm patients and cause additional workload for nurses and other clinicians.
- By advocating for strong usability testing methods by vendors and identifying usability problems, nurses can play a critical role in decreasing the technology associated workload and improving the technology's usefulness.

INTRODUCTION AND BACKGROUND

Technology in health care is now ubiquitous. Intensive Care Units, in particular, are a virtual sea of technology, often adding complexity to the environment where critically ill patients receive life-saving care. Nurses are often at the center of this complexity, using technologies[1] in their role of provider of hands-on care on behalf of the health care team. In addition to hands-on care, ICU nurses rely on clinical technologies to support one of their most important responsibilities: vigilance. That is, as the clinicians who spend the most time observing and assessing patients,[2] nurses play the primary role in detecting and responding to moment to moment clinical changes in critically ill patients to detect and respond rapidly to signs of patient deterioration.[3]

The authors have no commercial interests to report.
[a] Health Systems Science, University of Illinois at Chicago College of Nursing, 845 South Damen Avenue MC 802, Chicago IL 60612, USA; [b] Decatur Memorial Hospital, 2300 N. Edward Street, Decatur, IL 62526, USA
* Corresponding author.
E-mail address: kdunnL2@uic.edu

There are multiple technologies to support the delivery of patient care in ICUs, including lifesaving technologies, technologies that monitor patients' ever-changing clinical conditions, technologies to retrieve patient medications, and technologies to directly deliver medications directly into the body.[4] In addition, health records are also now technologies (electronic health records [EHRs]) that are designed to both retrieve patient information, communicate a patient's condition to the entire team, provide a safe mechanism to order and administer medications, and document interventions.[5]

EHRs likely represent a major source of increased complexity both in and outside ICUs[6] for a majority of practicing nurses. In an effort to make care safer, a federal law was enacted in 2009 that gave strong incentives to EHR adoption.[7] By 2015, 83.8% of nonfederal acute care hospitals in the United States had adopted an EHR.[8] EHRs are used by both large and small hospitals and, in 2016, hospitals with fewer than 200 beds accounted for 78% of EHR purchases.[9] Even hospitals with existing comprehensive EHRs were impacted by the federal law, because a large number of hospitals changed to federally compliant new systems. Other reasons prompting EHR change over the past several years include the formation of new strategic partnerships, instability in the smaller EHR vendor market, and changing organizational needs.[9] This means that a majority of nurses employed at hospitals not only currently work with an EHR but also they likely lived through a major EHR implementation.

The process of using EHRs and other technologies to make care safer has also added additional workload.[10,11] What in the past may have been opening a paper chart and writing a structured note using free-text now involves a multistep computer log-in, identifying the relevant patients EHR from a list, scanning a list of electronic tabs to find the right section, and a series of mouse scrolling and searching for appropriate checkboxes and data entry fields. In addition, many EHRs provide a newer type of technology: clinical decision support (CDS). CDS provides real-time computer-generated information about a patient within the EHR that assists nurses[12] (and other clinicians)[13] in making decisions[14] and adhering to evidence-based guidelines. Although CDS supports decision-making and evidence-based practice, it often adds additional steps and may even temporarily stop workflow. Given the wide range of technologies that ICU nurses must use, it is not surprising that technologies with different functions are often designed by different vendors. This generally means that the interface, use steps, audible alarms, and so forth differ from technology to technology, further adding to the complexity of technology use in ICUs.

These technologies are integral to providing health care in the digital age and have led to many positive outcomes related to patient safety.[15–18] Unfortunately technology does not prevent all patient harm and can even facilitate nursing errors.[19,20] There is evidence of serious unintended consequences from health information technologies.[21–24] These problems are serious and include alert fatigue,[25–27] administration of multiple does of the same medication[28] or the wrong medication,[15] difficulty determining which medications are due,[28] and omission of scheduled medication administration.[28]

Given the complexity, major system changes, additional workload, and unintended consequences, health care providers are increasingly frustrated with technologies they find difficult to use.[18,29] Excessive clicks needed to access information, confusing alerts, too many alerts, false-positive alarms, and so forth are often routine parts of a clinician's day. What may seem like a simple problem or a small extra step is now compounded by the number of tasks now mediated by computer and other technologies. With medical errors estimated to be the third leading cause of death[30] and burnout a problem in retaining well-trained staff,[31–33] it is imperative that nurses and other clinicians are engaged and empowered to influence the design and purchase of technologies that are highly usable and make it easier to provide safe and high-quality care.

OBJECTIVES

The purpose of this article is to (1) provide the needed usability, design, and testing vocabulary to identify and articulate clinical technology usability problems and (2) provide ideas on ways to advocate and impact positive change related to technology usability within a health care organization.

What Makes a Technology Usable and Useful?

A technology must have *usability* and *utility* to be considered useful. In the contest of technology usefulness, *utility* refers to whether a technology fits a need of users (people who potentially will use or are currently using a system, not the designers or programmers)—whether it does what it was designed to do. *Usability* refers to a quality that assesses how easy user interfaces are to use. It has been formally defined by the International Organization for Standardization as "The extent to which a product can be used by specified users to achieve specified goals with effectiveness, efficiency and satisfaction in a specified context of use."[34] Nielsen[35], a leader in the field of usability engineering, broadened and clarified the term further by defining 5 key components of usability: (1) efficient to use, (2) easy to learn, (3) easy to remember, (4) low error rate and easy error recovery, and (5) subjectively pleasing (**Table 1**).

Overview of Usability Assessment Methods

Assessment of a technology usability in health care is categorized in 4 major types conducted by vendors and researchers: (1) inspection methods, (2) formal usability testing, (3) summative testing, and (4) field studies.

Inspection method

After a preliminary design or functioning prototype (a model that is used to design the full system from), experts (human factors, engineers and clinical) should perform some kind of systematic inspection of the prototype to uncover usability problems. One

Table 1 Attributes of technology usefulness		
Concept	**Attribute**	**Definition**
Utility		Technologies that meet a user's need by correctly doing what they were designed to do
Usability	Efficient	Once a user has learned the system, the system allows the user to perform at a high productivity level.
	Learnable	Technologies that are so easy to learn that users can quickly perform the tasks the first time they interact with it
	Memorable	Technologies that are so easy to remember that a user can quickly recall how to perform tasks after a period of nonuse
	Errors	Prevention of catastrophic errors and easy recovery from errors
	Satisfaction	The technology is subjectively satisfying to the user.

Data from Nielsen J. What is usability? In: Nielsen J, editor. Usability engineering. San Diego: Academic Press; 1993. p. 23–48.

such example of this is called *heuristic evaluation*, which systematically evaluates the technology with known human computer interface design principles.[36] This evaluation usually focuses on 10 major factors[36,37]:

- **Visibility of system status**: the systems should include some kind of display that keeps users aware of what a system is doing. This is especially important when the system is searching for information and work in the system is temporarily paused.
- **Match between system and the real world**: the system should use words, phrases, and concepts that are familiar to the intended users.
- **User control and freedom**: the systems should have ways that the user can exit, undo, and redo.
- **Consistency and standards**: there should be consistency in words, colors, and icons throughout the system and when possible use conventions common outside the system (eg, red = stop).
- **Error prevention**: designs should prevent users from making errors from occurring (eg, limit systolic blood pressure data fields to 3 characters).
- **Recognition rather than recall**: designs should minimize the user's memory load by making instructions, actions, and options easily visible. This way users can recognize the way to use the system without taxing memory load to recall their training.
- **Flexibility and efficiency of use**: designs that allow different efficient means (eg, shortcuts) expert users can use to accomplish frequent tasks.
- **Aesthetic and minimalist design**: designs should not include extra information because every piece of additional information diminishes the visibility of essential information.
- **Help users recognize, diagnose, and recover from errors**: design should include error messages that indicate the problem and potential solutions in plain language that are clearly visible.
- **Help and documentation**: although the goal is that a system can be used without support, it is sometimes necessary to have easily accessible help documentation within the system.

Another inspection method is called *cognitive walkthrough*. Cognitive walkthrough is another common systematic procedure that focuses on how well the interface can be used without training.[5] Other methods combine the 2 approaches or focus on inspection of specific features.[3] Whichever inspection method is used, it is important for key members of the purchasing organization to know if some kind of systematic inspection was used before the technology is tested with potential users.

Formal usability testing

Usability testing refers to the evaluation of a technology or software system that involves tests by design and usability experts with a representative group of potential users of the technology as they perform tasks using the system.[38] Rather than conduct tests with large groups of users, repeated cycles with small numbers of testers (8–10) are often considered best practice for usability testing during the creation and refinement process[38] (often referred to as *formative testing*). The process of iteratively designing, called *user-centered design*, allows the vendors to identify problems and obtain feedback that can be iteratively incorporated into the design.[39] Using this method, vendors have the opportunity to substantially improve the usability and may be implementing a design that has been improved several times before implementation.

One common method is called the *think-aloud method*. Think-alouds are a simple and inexpensive method whereby future systems users test the system while narrating what they are doing and why they are doing it while interacting with the system to perform given tasks.[40] The moderator of the test does little speaking or question asking. Rather, moderators encourages test users to have a running dialogue of the thought processes so they can understand what motivated test users' actions that could be moving them toward an unintended decision (eg, "I see this little book symbol...not sure what it means, maybe it means there is important information...since most of my days are busy and this does not look important, I don't think I'm going to click it").

Analysis of think-alouds often involves a video recording that synchronizes test users' words with what they are seeing and interacting with on the screens, to pinpoint areas of the interface that were not used correctly or confused test users, in order to redesign.[40] Think-alouds are often conducted using clinical scenarios and some degree of clinical care simulation. They can be low fidelity, such as a computer laboratory where test users are given a clinical scenario and asked to make a decision in the way they would in clinical practice, or high fidelity, which can include a physical environment that emulates a clinical setting, clinical noises, and distractions and actors to portray patients and other members of the health care team.

Another method used less commonly, but valuable to the design of CDS, is called *cognitive interviewing*.[40] This method involves asking test users questions about how they interpret clinical alert messages. Clinician interpretations may not be apparent in a think-aloud interview and it is important to solicit test users' interpretations. For example, it is possible that what the designers intended to be a "call to action" for a nurse might be interpreted by a nurse as "something they can't really do anything about."

There are a variety of other usability testing methods available to vendors and easy-to-access evidence-based toolkits during the design and refinement process.[41,42] Unfortunately, a study of EHR vendors revealed that formal usability testing, user-centered design approaches, and employment of usability experts are rare.[43] In addition, some vendors may only test their system with nonclinician staff.[44] Therefore, it is critical for hospital administrators and nurses involved in the technology selection process to be assertive on this particular issue. Systems that have not been tested on representative users (eg, software to be sued by nurses is only tested by physicians) should be viewed negatively.

Summative testing

Summative testing (also referred to as *validation testing*) is done closer to the end of the design cycle once a majority of errors and usability problems have been detected.[42] This may be done in larger groups of potential users to allow for validation of the technology with statistical analysis. This round of testing may be done by the vendor or by objective researchers. The aims of this round of testing evaluate effectiveness but may also include usability questionnaires (such as the System Usability Scale)[45] and possible cognitive workload (such as National Aeronautics and Space Administration Task Load Index).[46,47]

Field studies

Qualitative methods or *field studies* conducted by experts in these methods and health care workflow or researchers are also important to determine usability. Conducted after the technology implementation, these structured (having a specific set of variables to examine) and unstructured (observers taking notes on anything they think would have the redesign process) observation methods of practice (eg, shadowing nurses as they work) are useful to uncover usability problems that were not deducted during laboratory test conditions.[21,28]

Remote testing

Testing usability can also be conducted by vendors or researchers with nurses and other clinicians using screen-sharing software.[48] Although this method is not featured prominently in the published literature, there are some vendors that rely on this method to improve usability. *Vendor remote testing* can be a valuable way for organizations to demonstrate clinician-identified usability problems to an EHR vendor and could be helpful for organizations with small information technology departments.

Virtual test environments

This type of testing, in simulated clinical conditions, can be done within health care organizations during the implementation of EHRs or to test new features within an existing EHR. A virtual test environment is created with scenarios meant to mimic real patient care at an institution. Generally, a team of clinician users are identified to walk through these scenarios and enter data simulating a patient flow through the hospital or clinic. Various disciplines participate to identify parts of the system that are not working correctly or missing pieces essential to the delivery of care in the particular care process being tested.

This type of testing can be labor intensive for an organization because experts in every area of the hospital are needed simultaneously to test these situations. The clinical informatics team solicits volunteers to do testing. Nurses can contact the clinical informatics team to express their interest in testing a new system. Although nurses who consider themselves "tech savvy" may be the first to volunteer, it is helpful to have testers who consider themselves "tech challenged" to identify a wider array of potential problems.

ASSESSING AND ADVOCATING FOR USABILITY WITHIN HEALTH CARE ORGANIZATIONS: WHAT CAN PRACTICING NURSES DO?

Although vendor and research usability testing may sound costly and time consuming, Nielsen[49] notes that many methods are simple and inexpensive and dubbed them "discount usability engineering." Some of these methods can be incorporated by non-engineers. Practicing nurses can play a valuable role at several points in the process, including the selection process, after system upgrades, after new features are added, and long after implementation.

Definitions and terms that allow nurses to articulate specific usability attributes and usability testing methods are discussed previously. This section describes several feasible ways nurses can participate in, provide data for, and advocate for usability improvements at the following times: before the initial go-live (that moment in time when the system is used during actual care delivery), during build (the vendor's process of compiling parts of the software program that are specific for the organization) and go-live, and in the months and years post–technology implementation.

Before Go-Live

Many hospitals identify end users early in the process for review of the software, dialogue with the vendors, and site visits to hospitals using the software under consideration. When that happens, it is time for nurses to volunteer, ask questions, and provide expert input. Many decisions are made prior to purchase as the project is defined and cost estimates are fine tuned. Some of the key questions that nurses involved in the purchasing decision should ask are shown in **Table 2**.

Table 2
Questions to ask about technology to identify usability problems

Concept	Attribute	Potential Questions
Utility		Does the technology do what nurses need it to do?
		Can tasks performed by nurses be more efficient and safe using the designed technology?
Usable	Efficient	Are there unneeded steps in the technology that if removed would not reduce the utility or safety?
	Learnable	Can a clinician learn to use the technology quickly?
		Are large technical manuals needed as reference?
	Memorable	How likely is it that a clinician could recall how to use the technology after a period of nonuse?
	Errors	What type of inspection methods (eg, heuristic evaluation) and usability tests did the vendor use to uncover potential errors?
	Satisfaction	Will clinicians enjoy using the technology?
		Will clinicians perceive the technology valuable to providing safe and high-quality care?
		What process does the vendor use to respond to usability problems that are identified after go-live?
Effective		Has summative testing to determine efficacy and usability been conducted?
		Were summative tests conducted by the vendor or by objective researchers?
		Have barriers to care delivery that could occur with a particular system given current workflows or patient populations been identified?
Vendor testing process		Determine usability methods that the vendor used when developing the EHR, including tests performed, types of experts, involvement of users (should be all types of workers that will use the EHR) during the design process, EHR tasks evaluated, and number of subjects.

Build and Go-Live

Once the purchase has been made, an extensive project plan is completed. Often systems come with best practice content that has been built to serve as a template for implementation. That prebuild content can be used as a base to design the EHR, but additional work with hospital subject matter experts is necessary to insure that the needs of particular patient populations are addressed and that unique workflows are identified in each care setting. For instance, the documentation for patients in a critical care unit where adult neurosurgery patients receive care may be significantly different from one where adult and pediatric cardiac patients are treated. Nurses who obtain all laboratory specimens for their patients have a different workflow from nurses who use a phlebotomy service to obtain specimens. Hospitals and software companies use a variety of techniques to build this customized content. There may be clinical informatics nurse specialists in the organization along with computer analysts who get specialized training in the build. If so, this could be a new career opportunity for practicing nurses who want to focus in the area of informatics. In other instances, outside experts do the build. Either way, the team involved in the build needs clinical input to understand workflows, special populations, roles, and duties of each member of the care team. Many organizations identify superusers for this step in the process and provide them with early training so they can help guide the build and be ready to help their peers during implementation.[50] A superuser can have a great deal of influence during the build phase and gains proficiency prior to using the system during care delivery.

Training and Go-Live

Prior to implementation of an EHR, nurses are offered training on the system. This training should be designed to allow practice in the specific workflows that will be important when the system is actually used to document patient care. Taking full advantage of all training and practice is a must. Often, several guided training opportunities are available as well as "learn at your own pace" practice sessions. It is essential to allow sufficient time for nurses to become familiar and proficient on the parts of the system before the go-live date. Almost as important, other members of the care team may need to be encouraged to complete the training in advance of go-live. This is critical to nursing practice, because physicians who do not receive training and cannot enter orders when EHRs go live will have a negative impact on practice.

For go-live, some hospitals choose a system-wide approach for implementation and others turn the system on 1 unit or department at a time. Both methods have benefits and challenges. Starting 1 unit or department at a time may seem to be the easiest implementation approach, but because patients are treated across a broad continuum of care and staff function in multiple practice areas, using 2 systems of documentation during a transition period within an organization can be challenging for administrators. For example, laboratory, pharmacy, dietary, and radiology departments often must be an all-or-nothing implementation. Because these departments cross all areas of practice, many hospitals choose an enterprise-wide implementation over the more gradual department-by-department or unit-by-unit roll-out.

TESTING IN CONTROLLED CLINICAL CONDITIONS WITHIN A HEALTH CARE ORGANIZATION
Nurse Practice Councils and Other Committees

Practice councils, working with clinical informatics specialists, can develop new workflows, new alerts and reminders, and new care planning content to constantly improve care at the bedside. While practice councils may be easily identifiable, to find other clinical information specialist you may need to ask questions to identify other people in the organization who are able to make changes in the system. Dialogue with those people, often clinical informatics nurses, helps them understand specific clinical practice and address ways the technology can be used effectively to support that practice. Usability issues can be addressed more rapidly with this type of partnership, allowing clinical nurses to realize the full potential of the available technology.

In addition, health care systems often have a committee structure where requested changes are vetted to determine if the change is possible and if it will have a positive impact. Additions and future upgrade options often surface in these committees, and priorities are set based on their recommendations. This committee structure can be complex in large organizations with multiple hospitals and clinics, but nurses who communicate to leadership about their desire to be involved in these committees can have a seat at the table when priorities for change are determined.

SUMMARY

Technologies are, and will be for the foreseeable future, central to the work of intensive care nurses. These technologies must be highly usable to ensure high-quality and safe care delivery without unnecessary increases in workload. Importantly when nurses, the frontline users of many patient care technologies, have a hunch that something is not working quite right with a technology or that a technology could be made easier, they can play an important role leading to system improvement. Change is possible with an increasing number of practicing nurses who are educated about what usability is, how to assess usability vendors' practices, and evidence-based design principles and who are empowered to advocate for changes.

REFERENCES

1. Tunlind A, Granström J, Engström Å. Nursing care in a high-technological environment: experiences of critical care nurses. Intensive Crit Care Nurs 2015; 31(2):116–23.
2. Alastalo M, Salminen L, Lakanmaa R-L, et al. Seeing beyond monitors—critical care nurses' multiple skills in patient observation: descriptive qualitative study. Intensive Crit Care Nurs 2017;42:80–7.
3. Adam S, Dawson D. The critical care continuum. In: Adam S, Osborne S, Welch J, editors. Critical care nursing. Oxford (United Kingdom): Oxford University Press; 2017. p. 1–2.
4. De Georgia MA, Kaffashi F, Jacono FJ, et al. Information technology in critical care: review of monitoring and data acquisition systems for patient care and research. ScientificWorldJournal 2015;2015:727694.
5. Office of the National Coordinator for Health Information Technology. Benefits of electronic health records. 2015. Available at: https://www.healthit.gov/providers-professionals/benefits-electronic-health-records-ehrs. Accessed October 11, 2017.
6. Harrington L, Kennerly D, Johnson C. Safety issues related to the electronic medical record (EMR): synthesis of the literature from the last decade, 2000-2009. J Healthc Manag 2011;56(1):31–44.
7. Health Information Technology for Economic and Clinical Health (HITECH) Act, 2009.
8. Henry J, Pylypchuk Y, Searcy T, et al. Adoption of electronic health record systems among US non-federal acute care hospitals: 2008-2015. Washington, DC: The Office of National Coordinator for Health Information Technology; 2016.
9. Bermudez E, Warburton P. Hospital EMR market share 2017: decision energy shifts to the small market. 2017. Available at: www.KLASresearch.com:.
10. Ash JS, Sittig DF, Poon EG, et al. The extent and importance of unintended consequences related to computerized provider order entry. J Am Med Inform Assoc 2007;14(4):415–23.
11. Ahmed A, Chandra S, Herasevich V, et al. The effect of two different electronic health record user interfaces on intensive care provider task load, errors of cognition, and performance. Crit Care Med 2011;39(7):1626–34.
12. Dunn Lopez K, Gephart SM, Raszewski R, et al. Integrative review of clinical decision support for registered nurses in acute care settings. J Am Med Inform Assoc 2017;24(2):441–50.
13. Bright TJ, Wong A, Dhurjati R, et al. Effect of clinical decision-support systemsa systematic review. Ann Intern Med 2012;157(1):29–43.
14. Teich JM, Osheroff JA, Pifer EA, et al. Clinical decision support in electronic prescribing: recommendations and an action plan: report of the joint clinical decision support workgroup. J Am Med Inform Assoc 2005;12(4):365–76.
15. Carayon P, Wetterneck TB, Cartmill R, et al. Medication safety in two intensive care units of a community teaching hospital after electronic health record

implementation: sociotechnical and human factors engineering considerations. J Patient Saf 2017. [Epub ahead of print].

16. Han JE, Rabinovich M, Abraham P, et al. Effect of electronic health record implementation in critical care on survival and medication errors. Am J Med Sci 2016; 351(6):576–81.

17. Ohashi K, Dalleur O, Dykes PC, et al. Benefits and risks of using smart pumps to reduce medication error rates: a systematic review. Drug Saf 2014;37(12): 1011–20.

18. Shanafelt TD, Dyrbye LN, Sinsky C, et al. Relationship between clerical burden and characteristics of the electronic environment with physician burnout and professional satisfaction. Paper presented at: Mayo Clinic Proceedings 2016.

19. Meeks DW, Smith MW, Taylor L, et al. An analysis of electronic health record-related patient safety concerns. J Am Med Inform Assoc 2014;21(6):1053–9.

20. Bagherian B, Mirzaei T, Sabzevari S, et al. Caring within a web of paradoxes: the critical care nurses' experiences of beneficial and harmful effects of technology on Nursing Care. 2016.

21. Koppel R, Wetterneck T, Telles JL, et al. Workarounds to barcode medication administration systems: their occurrences, causes, and threats to patient safety. J Am Med Inform Assoc 2008;15(4):408–23.

22. Spetz J, Burgess JF, Phibbs CS. The effect of health information technology implementation in Veterans Health Administration hospitals on patient outcomes. Paper presented at: Healthcare 2014.

23. Han YY, Carcillo JA, Venkataraman ST, et al. Unexpected increased mortality after implementation of a commercially sold computerized physician order entry system. Pediatrics 2005;116(6):1506–12.

24. Un-named. Computer glitch may have led to incorrect prescription of statins. The Guardian 2016.

25. Gazarian PK. Nurses' response to frequency and types of electrocardiography alarms in a non-critical care setting: a descriptive study. Int J Nurs Stud 2014; 51(2):190–7.

26. Carspecken CW, Sharek PJ, Longhurst C, et al. A clinical case of electronic health record drug alert fatigue: consequences for patient outcome. Pediatrics 2013;131(6):e1970–3.

27. Embi PJ, Leonard AC. Evaluating alert fatigue over time to EHR-based clinical trial alerts: findings from a randomized controlled study. J Am Med Inform Assoc 2012;19(e1):e145–8.

28. Guo J, Iribarren S, Kapsandoy S, et al. Usability evaluation of an electronic medication administration record (eMAR) application. Appl Clin Inform 2011;2(2): 202–24.

29. Kruse CS, Argueta DA, Lopez L, et al. Patient and provider attitudes toward the use of patient portals for the management of chronic disease: a systematic review. J Med Internet Res 2015;17:e40.

30. Makary MA, Daniel M. Medical error-the third leading cause of death in the US. BMJ 2016;353:i2139.

31. Vargas C, Cañadas GA, Aguayo R, et al. Which occupational risk factors are associated with burnout in nursing? A meta-analytic study. Int J Clin Health Psychol 2014;14(1):28–38.

32. Dall'Ora C, Griffiths P, Ball J, et al. Association of 12 h shifts and nurses' job satisfaction, burnout and intention to leave: findings from a cross-sectional study of 12 European countries. BMJ Open 2015;5(9):e008331.

33. Dyrbye LN, Shanafelt TD, Sinsky CA, et al. Burnout among health care profes-
    sionals: a call to explore and address this underrecognized threat to safe,
    high-quality care. NAM (National Academy of Medicine) Perspectives; 2017.
34. Organization IS. Ergonomic requirements for office work with visual display termi-
    nals (VDTs) — Part 11: guidance on usability. Vol ISO 9241–11:19981998.
35. Nielsen J. What is usability?. In: Nielsen J, editor. Usability engineering. San
    Diego (CA): Academic Press; 1993. p. 23–37.
36. Nielsen J. Usability heuristics. In: Nielsen J, editor. Usability engineering. San
    Diego (CA): Academic Press; 1993. p. 115–55.
37. Usability.gov. Heurstic evaluations and expert reviews. 2017. Available at: https://
    www.usability.gov/how-to-and-tools/methods/heuristic-evaluation.html. Accessed
    October 5, 2017.
38. Kushniruk AW, Patel VL. Cognitive and usability engineering methods for the eval-
    uation of clinical information systems. J Biomed Inform 2004;37(1):56–76.
39. Usability.gov. User-centered design basics. What & why of usability. 2017. Avail-
    able at: https://www.usability.gov/what-and-why/user-centered-design.html.
40. Lopez KD, Febretti A, Stifter J, et al. Toward a more robust and efficient usability
    testing method of clinical decision support for nurses derived from nursing elec-
    tronic health record data. Int J Nurs knowl 2017;28(4):211–8.
41. Usability.gov. Usability glossary. What and why of usability. 2017. Available at:
    https://www.usability.gov/what-and-why/glossary/c/index.html.
42. Lowry SZ, Quinn MT, Ramaiah M, et al. Technical evaluation, testing, and valida-
    tion of the usability of electronic health records. Gaithersburg (MD): National Insti-
    tute of Standards and Technology; 2012. p. 65–87.
43. McDonnell C, Werner K, Wendel L. Electronic health record usability: vendor
    practices and perspectives. AHRQ; 2010.
44. Ratwani RM, Fairbanks RJ, Hettinger AZ, et al. Electronic health record usability:
    analysis of the user-centered design processes of eleven electronic health record
    vendors. J Am Med Inform Assoc 2015;22(6):1179–82.
45. Sousa VE, Lopez KD. Towards usable e-health. Appl Clin Inform 2017;8(2):
    470–90.
46. Colligan L, Potts HW, Finn CT, et al. Cognitive workload changes for nurses tran-
    sitioning from a legacy system with paper documentation to a commercial elec-
    tronic health record. Int J Med Inform 2015;84(7):469–76.
47. Administration NAaS. NASA Task Load Index. 2017. Available at: https://
    humansystems.arc.nasa.gov/groups/tlx/. Accessed October 31, 2017.
48. Usability.gov. Remote testing. How to & tools 2017. Available at: https://www.
    usability.gov/how-to-and-tools/methods/remote-testing.html.
49. Nielsen J. Discount usability engineering. In: Usability engineering. San Diego:
    Academic press; 1993. p. 17–20.
50. Yuan CT, Bradley EH, Nembhard IM. A mixed methods study of how clinician
    'super users' influence others during the implementation of electronic health re-
    cords. BMC Med Inform Decis Mak 2015;15:26.

Work System Barriers and Strategies Reported by Tele-Intensive Care Unit Nurses
A Case Study

Peter L.T. Hoonakker, PhD[a],*, Pascale Carayon, PhD[b]

KEYWORDS

• Virtual teams • Dynamic relationships • Intensive care units • Tele-medicine

KEY POINTS

• There is a shortage of intensive care personnel, both intensivists and critical nurses.
• This shortage can partly be remediated by implementation of tele-intensive care units (ICUs).
• The literature shows that tele-ICUs can have several benefits, but that the virtual collaboration between personnel in the ICUs that are monitored and the tele-ICU can be difficult.
• Tele-ICU nurses have to deal with many different hospitals, ICUs, ICU staff, health information technology, medical devices and protocols, which makes their jobs difficult.
• This lack of familiarity can cause all kind of barriers and tele-ICU nurses have to develop strategies to manage these barriers.

INTRODUCTION

Intensive care units (ICUs) are highly complex organizations where lives are hanging by a thread. Approximately 400,000 to 500,000 people die each year in American ICUs.[1,2] The highly complex environment and great responsibilities put a burden on

Disclosure Statement: The authors have no conflict of interest.
This study was made possible with support from the National Science Foundation (NSF Grant #: OCI-0838513, PI: P. Carayon, and NSF grant # CMMI 1536987, PI: Li) and the cooperation from the manager and the nurses who work in the tele-ICU.
Funded by: NIH. Grant number(s): NIH National Center for Advancing Translational Sciences, grant UL1TR002373; NIHMS-ID: 942520.
[a] Center for Quality and Productivity Improvement, University of Wisconsin-Madison, 3124 Engineering Centers Building, 1550 Engineering Drive, Madison, WI 53706, USA; [b] Department of Industrial and Systems Engineering, Center for Quality and Productivity Improvement, University of Wisconsin-Madison, 3126 Engineering Centers Building, 1550 Engineering Drive, Madison, WI 53706, USA
* Corresponding author.
E-mail address: Peter.Hoonakker@wisc.edu

ICU staff. There is a shortage of ICU personnel,[3–7] and in the past decades, the number of critical care beds has increased, whereas the number of hospitals offering critical care services has decreased. Tele-ICUs may be a solution for the shortage of ICU personnel. In a tele-ICU, patients are monitored remotely by physicians and nurses trained in critical care. A tele-ICU nurse can monitor up to as many as 50 ICU patients in different ICUs and hospitals. Tele-ICU nurses use the most recent technology that provides access to patient information as well as video and audio links to patient rooms. Tele-ICU physicians and nurses collaborate with physicians and nurses in the ICUs in what can be considered virtual teams.

We know little about the collaboration between staff in the tele-ICU and ICUs in this type of virtual team. Tele-ICUs are virtual teams that pose unique challenges because of their dynamic and fluid membership: tele-ICU nurses and physicians have to deal with many ICUs simultaneously.[8] In this article, we describe the work system barriers experienced by tele-ICU nurses and identify strategies tele-ICU nurses use in dealing with these barriers. We also explore the negative or positive consequences of strategies.

BACKGROUND

Tele-ICUs are units where intensivists and nurses provide 24/7 care, support, and advice from a distance to remote ICUs. Various forms of health information technology are used to support the sharing of information between the tele-ICU and the ICUs. Technologies allow tele-ICU intensivists and nurses to monitor patients, to observe patients and medical devices in the patient room though a camera, and to communicate with ICU nurses and providers. Several studies provide a detailed description of the evolution of the tele-ICU, the tele-ICU organization, and tele-ICU nurses' activities.[3,7,9–13] Tele-ICUs are a relatively new phenomenon; the "oldest" tele-ICU has been in existence for more than 15 years.[3] Nearly 10% of patients in American ICUs are currently monitored by tele-ICUs.[9]

The tele-ICU team can be composed of multiple clinicians: board-certified intensivists, critical care nurses, clerical personnel, and, in some instances, a pharmacist. Personnel in the ICU (including residents on duty in the ICU) receive instructions or guidance from the tele-ICU staff and may have the opportunity to learn new skills and knowledge.[14] Tele-monitoring is crucial to the tele-ICU model. Personnel in the tele-ICU receive patient data in real time and, therefore, can detect trends in patient status; they can then alert personnel in the ICU.[15]

Tele-ICU physicians and nurses work at workstations that are commonly composed of multiple monitors, a 2-way camera, microphone, and a high-speed dial phone. Clinical data captured about the ICU patient are directly streamed to the tele-ICU. Tele-ICU clinicians depend on information communicated over the phone or entered into the computer from the bedside to inform them on the current state of the patient. They monitor numerous clinical indicators, such as blood pressure, heart rate, ventilator settings, and oxygen saturation. Other data such as patient care plans, laboratory results, and radiographs are send electronically or faxed to the tele-ICU. Most tele-ICU software uses "smart alarms" to alert the clinicians to possible significant changes in patient status.

Tele-Intensive Care Unit Literature

Most studies on the tele-ICU have focused on clinical and financial outcomes.[16–22] Several studies have reported that the implementation of an ICU telemedicine program can improve clinical care outcomes (eg, reduced duration of stay, reduced mortality, reduced complications) and reduce health care costs.[16,19–24] However, other studies have failed to confirm some of these positive outcomes.[25–28]

The study by Anders and colleagues[15] focused on the functions of the tele-ICU. The researchers performed 40 hours of observation of 8 tele-ICU nurses and 1 tele-ICU physician in 1 tele-ICU. Results showed that the tele-ICU fulfills 3 functions: (1) anomaly response—tele-ICU nurses processed information related to alerts and alarms and contacted other staff in the tele-ICU or the ICU if they perceived the need for follow-up or action; (2) access to specialized expertise—experienced tele-ICU nurses were observed to mentor junior ICU nurses; ICU nurses had access to expertise and experience of the tele-ICU nurses thereby augmenting their knowledge base; and (3) sense making—tele-ICU nurses can make sense of what is happening with patients because they have access to many sources of data and have the resources (time, expertise) to synthesize the data. Research on tele-ICUs is limited; in particular nursing issues related to tele-ICU have been overlooked.[29] Few studies have explored how tele-ICU nurses deal with multiple interactions across varied ICUs and hospitals.[30,31] We need to know more about the work system barriers experienced by tele-ICU nurses, as well as the strategies they use to deal with these barriers and their consequences.

METHODS
Study Design

We used a case study design to investigate work system barriers experienced by tele-ICU nurses and the strategies they use to manage multiple ICUs.[32,33] A case study is a research strategy and an empirical inquiry that investigates a phenomenon within its real-life context, using multiple data collection instruments. We used various methods (observations, interviews, surveys, and field notes) to collect data in the tele-ICU. In this article, we focus on the analysis of interview data.

Setting and Sample

The participating tele-ICU has been in existence since 2003 and monitors 260 beds in 15 ICUs of 6 different hospitals. The tele-ICU employs totally 42 nurses and 20 physicians in different shifts. On average, a tele-ICU nurse monitors 45 beds. We interviewed 10 tele-ICU nurses who volunteered to participate in the study.

Data Collection Instrument

We used a semistructured interview guide (see http://cqpi.wisc.edu/wp-uploads/2016/07/Tele-ICU_Nurse_Interview_Guide.pdf for the interview guide). The interviews addressed the following topics: a typical day in the tele-ICU, tools and software used, interaction with multiple ICUs, how to deal with crisis situations, communication between tele-ICU and ICU, relationship with ICUs, trust in relationships with ICUs, and quality of care. In this article, we examine work system barriers experienced by tele-ICU nurses in dealing with multiple ICUs. The questions asked included: "What are the challenges of interacting with multiple ICUs?" We used additional prompts such as: "Why is it easy? – Could you give us specific examples?" and "Why is it difficult? – Could you give us specific examples?" The interviews lasted about 1 hour. Interviews were audio-recorded, transcribed, and made anonymous to protect confidentiality of the interviewees. The study was approved by the Institutional Review Board of the University of Wisconsin—Madison.

Data Analysis

Interview data were analyzed using the qualitative data analysis NVivo software (QSR International, Melbourne, Australia). The transcripts of the interviews were imported in NVivo and were coded to answer the research question. We took several steps to analyze the data. First, we identified barriers and strategies used by tele-ICU nurses to deal with the barriers. This initial coding was performed on 2 interview transcripts. Over several team meetings, we discussed the coding, and began to create nodes (major categories of interview text based on their content similarities and unique relationships) for the 3 major topics related to our research objective: work system barriers, strategies to deal with the barriers, and consequences of the strategies. The researchers then coded the text in NVivo and identified barriers, strategies and consequences, while keeping track of the nodes, their definitions and examples. Finally, we created 3 matrices to link (1) barriers and strategies, (2) strategies and consequences, and (3) barriers and consequences. We also computed frequencies for each barrier, strategy, and consequence. When a nurse mentioned a specific topic several times during the interview, the topic was counted as 1. The minimum number of times a topic is mentioned is 1 (1 nurse); and the maximum is 10 (10 nurses mentioned it).

RESULTS

Barriers

The 10 tele-ICU nurses mentioned a total of 166 barriers in dealing with multiple ICUs. The barriers were categorized in 6 main categories: barriers with regard to the particular characteristics of the different ICUs, barriers with regard to patient care, barriers with regard to the relationship between the ICUs and the tele-ICU, barriers with regard to the technology, barriers associated with the organization of the tele-ICU, and barriers in the tasks of tele-ICU nurses. Results are summarized in **Table 1**.

Strategies

Tele-ICU nurses mentioned 98 instances of strategies in dealing with the barriers; those were categorized in 14 major strategies. **Table 2** presents the data for strategies.

Consequences

Although we did not explicitly ask about the possible consequences of dealing with barriers in interacting with multiple ICUs, nurses reported a total of 25 instances of consequence that were categorized into 12 major categories (**Table 3**).

Relationships Between Barriers, Strategies, and Consequences in Interacting with Multiple Intensive Care Units

The relationships between barriers, strategies, and consequences are displayed in **Fig. 1**. Only the main data are shown in **Fig. 1** to facilitate reading and comprehension of the graph. Barriers were included if they were mentioned by at least 5 tele-ICU nurses, strategies if they were mentioned by at least 4 nurses; and consequences if they were mentioned by at least 2 nurses. Relationships between barriers and strategies were included if they were mentioned by at least 3 nurses.

DISCUSSION

The results of our analyses on the barriers experienced by tele-ICU nurses in managing multiple ICUs show a range of barriers, strategies, and consequences. Most comments about barriers concern the relationship of the tele-ICU with the ICUs (see **Table 1**). A lot of ambiguity and sometimes conflict can occur because the ICUs are not familiar with the tele-ICU and its staff or do not understand the purpose of tele-ICU (mentioned by 10 nurses). We also found limited trust between the tele-ICU

Table 1
Barriers reported by tele-ICU nurses

Barriers	Examples	No. of Nurses
Barriers related to characteristics of the ICUs		
Variety of ICUs	Different ICUs have different characteristics and differences in the way work is organized.	7
Variety in ICU care processes	Different ICUs have different patient care processes and protocols.	6
Variety of ICU staff	Different ICU clinicians have different personalities, behaviors and characteristics.	8
Limited ICU nurse experience	ICU RNs have limited experience in the ICU.	5
Barriers with regard to patient, patient information and patient care issues		
Lack of and poor access to patient-related information	The tele-ICU RN has limited access to patient-related information or cannot find patient-related information.	3
Lack of care for patient from ICUs	ICU may be too busy with one patient and may not be able to provide care to the other patient.	2
Lack of knowledge of patient	The tele-ICU RN has limited knowledge or not the most up-to-date patient information about a patient.	7
Lack of or poor documentation	Documentation on patient care is lacking or poor.	6
Barriers in the relationship between tele-ICU and ICU		
ICU's lack of familiarity with tele-ICU staff and purpose	ICU staff has lack of familiarity with tele-ICU staff and the purpose of the tele-ICU.	10
Lack of acceptance of tele-ICU	The ICU clinicians do not accept the tele-ICU, do not want to work with the tele-ICU, and do not see value of the tele-ICU.	9
Lack of or poor communication with ICU	The communication between the tele-ICU RN and ICU staff is limited or poor.	6
Lack of familiarity with ICU staff	The tele-ICU RN is not familiar with the ICU staff.	9
Lack of or variety of trust between tele-ICU and ICU	There is a variety in trust from tele-ICU to ICUs and vice versa.	8
Tele-ICU RN has lack of awareness regarding of what is happening in ICUs	Tele-ICU RN does not know what is going on in the ICU. For example, how busy the ICU is or the workload of the ICU RNs.	5
Variety in acceptance and use of tele-ICU	There are differences in level of acceptance and use of the tele-ICU by the ICUs. Some ICUs need the tele-ICU more than others.	9
Conflict with ICU	The tele-ICU RN has a different opinion about patient care than ICU staff.	6

(continued on next page)

Table 1 (*continued*)		
Barriers	**Examples**	**No. of Nurses**
Barriers with regard to the technology (equipment, devices, or health information technology)		
Lack of familiarity with and knowledge of ICU equipment or devices	The tele-ICU RN does not know or is not familiar with ICU equipment and devices (eg, ventilator, infusion pump, and monitors).	6
Problem with tele-ICU equipment or software	ICUs do not use tele-ICU software to document because ICUs have lack of familiarity with tele-ICU software such as VISICU software.	5
General IT problems	Tele-ICU RN has problem with IT, either with tele-ICU equipment/software or other IT problem(s).	2
Barriers with regard to the organization and characteristics of the tele-ICU		
Variation in ICU assignment	The tele-ICU RN gets assigned to different ICUs for each shift.	2
Variation of tele-ICU staff, work styles and personalities	The clinicians in the tele-ICU have a variety of personalities and the tele-ICU RN has to learn to work with different personalities.	2
Barriers with regard to the job or task design of tele-ICU nurses		
Cognitive or memory load	The tele-ICU RN has to remember different things, including ways of login into EHR, passwords, and way to access information.	9
High workload	The tele-ICU RN experiences high workload, for example, because of the number of admissions, demands from multiple ICU staff, and insufficient staff coverage.	10
Interruption(s)	The tele-ICU RN is interrupted when performing his or her tasks.	9
Staying vigilant	It is hard for tele-ICU RN to stay alert and awake, and maintain attention after prolonged periods in his or her shift.	3
Uncertainty	The tele-ICU RN experiences uncertainty with regard to what will happen next.	3

Abbreviations: EHR, electronic health record; ICU, intensive care unit; IT, information technology; RN, registered nurse.

and the ICUs (n = 8), limited acceptance and use of the tele-ICU by the ICUs (n = 9), and, on the tele-ICU side, a lack of familiarity with staff in the different ICUs. All of this can result in poor communication (n = 6) and even conflict (n = 6).

A second major category of barriers is created by the large diversity in the different ICUs monitored by tele-ICU nurses. The tele-ICU monitors a total of 15 ICUs in 6 different hospitals. This variety in ICUs (mentioned 7 times) implies that tele-ICU nurses deal with a large variety of ICU staff (n = 8), variety in the experience of ICU nurses (n = 5), and a variety of ICU protocols and care processes (n = 6). The tele-ICU nurses, although all trained as ICU nurses themselves, often have limited experience in some types of ICUs (eg, cardiac ICU in an urban hospital). Tele-ICU nurses

Table 2
Strategies used by tele-ICU nurses in dealing with barriers

#	Strategies	Description	No. of Nurses
1	Adapt to ICU	The tele-ICU nurse has to adapt the way they deal with ICU staff, so they can be more receptive to the tele-ICU.	7
2	Anticipate or prevent problems	Tele-ICU nurse anticipate problem and take action to prevent problems.	8
3	Ask for (additional) information	The tele-nurse asks for (additional or specific) information from ICU staff to assess changes in patient conditions, ICU protocols, ICU equipment, when tele-ICU nurse cannot find information on the flow sheet.	7
4	Ask for support	The tele-ICU nurse asks for help and support from their colleagues in the tele-ICU to handle multiple ICUs.	9
5	Check information	The tele-ICU nurse checks to make sure that the patient information that she or he has is correct.	4
6	Facilitate communication	The tele-ICU nurse performs actions that may improve relationships and communications with ICUs.	10
7	Figure out	The tele-ICU nurse tries to figure out how to work with different ICUs, different EHRs and different ICU nurses (ie, how to communicate with them).	6
8	Obtain and search for (additional) information	The tele-ICU nurse obtains and searches for (additional) patient related information without interacting with ICU staff.	8
9	Organize information and tasks	The tele-ICU nurse better organizes the available patient information to help him or her deal with multiple patients. For example, tele-ICU nurse uses paper notes to keep track of patient, uses a mental checklist to remember what to come back to after getting interrupted.	10
10	Prioritize	The tele-ICU nurse makes active decisions on what problem to tackle first. For example, when there are a lot of admissions, tele-ICU nurse needs to prioritize which patient to handle first.	4
11	Provide support	The tele-ICU nurse provides informational or emotional support to ICU nurses or tele-ICU nurses to help them taking care of patients.	10
12	Share information	The tele-ICU nurse shares information (such as standardized protocol) with ICUs.	4
13	Take little or no action	The tele-ICU nurse does not interact with ICU nurses because of lack of ICU acceptance.	4
14	Workaround problem	The tele-ICU nurse works around the problem. For example, the tele-ICU nurse uses password cheat sheets to help him or her remember the passwords, the tele-ICU nurse tricks the system to log in	9

Abbreviation: ICU, intensive care unit.

Table 3
Consequences of dealing with barriers experienced by tele-ICU nurses

#	Consequences	Description	No. of Nurses
1	Additional workload	The tele-ICU RN experiences additional workload.	1
2	Delay in patient care	Care provided to an ICU patient is delayed (eg, delay in assistance, delay in switching between patients).	1
3	Error	Tele-ICU RN makes error when she deals with multiple ICUs. For example, tele-ICU RN entered information into the wrong patient chart or missed alerts.	1
4	Improved patient care	The care provided to the ICU patient is improved.	1
5	Improved relationship between tele-ICU and ICU	The relationship between the tele-ICU and ICU is improved (eg, more information provided, experience of RN aids credibility).	5
6	Increased knowledge about patient by tele-ICU	The tele-ICU RN has additional knowledge about the patient, for example, because of increased communication with the ICU.	1
7	No impact on patient care	There is no impact on care provided to the ICU patient	1
8	Poor communication	Communication between the ICU and tele-ICU RN is negatively affected.	1
9	Feeling bad	Tele-ICU RN feels bad about her work in the tele-ICU or bad because of lack of acceptance by ICU RN.	3
10	Frustrating	Frustration is experienced by the tele-ICU RN.	4
11	Stressful	Stress is experienced by the tele-ICU RN.	3
12	Time consuming	The tele-ICU spends more time performing tasks (eg, finding information, navigating systems, logging in).	1

Abbreviations: ICU, intensive care unit; RN, registered nurse.

have to deal with different kinds of hospitals (teaching, academic, etc) and different ICUs (open and closed ICUs, cardiac, medical, surgical, neurologic, special, etc) within these hospitals. Apart from differences in ICU type, ICUs may have different care processes, protocols, health information technology applications, and medical devices. All of these differences can, on the one hand, be an interesting challenge and provide opportunities for tele-ICU nurses to learn new things; but, on the other hand, these differences can be confusing.[34]

A third major barrier in the interaction with multiple ICUs is the way the job of a tele-ICU nurse is designed. Tele-ICU nurses mention high mental workload (n = 10), have occasional problems with the long 12-hour shifts that require them to stay vigilant for a long time (n = 3), and are often interrupted in their activities (n = 9). Tele-ICU nurses can monitor up to 50 ICU patients, and are often interrupted with requests from (nurses in) the ICUs that they monitor, and from colleagues (both physicians and nurses) in the tele-ICU. Part of the high workload is the large volume of patients being admitted and discharged. That makes it sometimes difficult to keep track of what is happening with patients and contribute to high cognitive workload (n = 9).

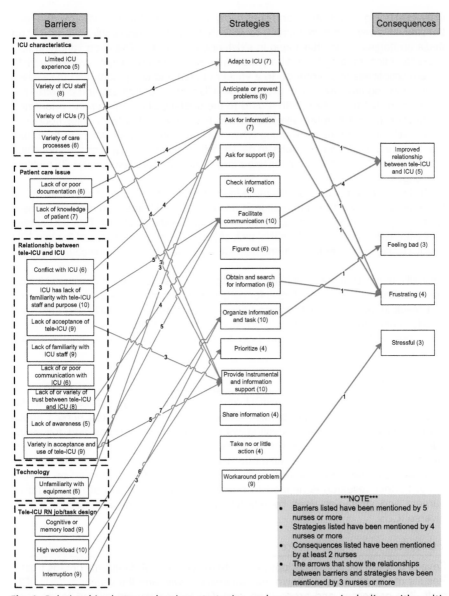

Fig. 1. Relationships between barriers, strategies, and consequences in dealing with multiple intensive care units (ICUs).

Tele-ICU nurses developed a wide range of strategies to deal with the different barriers (see **Table 2**). We linked the strategies to barriers (see **Fig. 1**). Tele-ICU nurses "react" to barriers using different strategies, for example, by facilitating communication, providing support, organizing information, and asking for or finding additional information.

Evidently, if tele-ICU nurses can facilitate communication with the ICUs, this strategy can help in reducing or mitigating problems with the relationship with the ICUs.[8,35] If the ICU staff realizes that the tele-ICU is there to help and assist them, instead of being "Big Brother" and controlling what they do, that may improve the relationship.[7] However, it is interesting to note that tele-ICU nurses still have to rely on these strategies, even after being in existence for 6 years. The large variety in ICU characteristics, ranging from differences in perspectives on patient care to a variety in care processes and protocols to a variety of staff and equipment, and the subsequent high cognitive workload, prompt tele-ICU nurses to organize and prioritize the information that they need. With regard to the strategy of organizing and prioritizing information (n = 10), most tele-ICU nurses use paper notes (with color codes) to keep track of what they were doing when they were interrupted. Many of them use these paper notes for the handoffs. In dealing with simultaneous dynamic relationships with multiple ICUs, tele-ICU nurses use a large range of strategies to deal with multiple challenges.

Strategies are often helpful with more than one type of barriers. As shown in **Fig. 1**, the strategy of asking for information is used by tele-ICU nurses to mitigate barriers related to patient care issues as well as unfamiliarity with equipment. Tele-ICU nurses deal with barriers related to the ICUs' lack of familiarity and knowledge of the tele-ICU and ICUs' lack of acceptance of the tele-ICU by engaging in communication with the ICUs.

Finally, tele-ICU nurses mentioned a number of consequences of dealing with barriers (see **Table 3**). When strategies for certain problems are successful, this outcome can result in improved relationships between the tele-ICU and ICUs and improved quality of care and patient safety.[14] However, when tele-ICU nurses cannot successfully cope with barriers, this can lead to frustration, stress, and other negative feelings.[7,8]

Study Limitations

This study took place in 1 tele-ICU and, therefore, the generalizability of the results is limited. During the semistructured interviews, we asked nurses about barriers they experienced in dealing with multiple ICUs. Probes and follow-up questions were used to ask nurses about how they dealt with strategies, but we did not explicitly and consistently ask them about potential consequences or outcomes. Therefore, data on consequences should be considered as exploratory. Further research is needed to deepen our understanding of the impact of barriers and strategies used by tele-ICU nurses to manage a large number of diverse ICUs.

Implications for Nursing Practice

Several of these recommendations pertain to the concept of "familiarity breeds trust." Results of this study have shown that unfamiliarity with and the variety in ICUs, ICU staff, ICU processes and procedures, and ICU technology are related to many of the barriers in the work of a tele-ICU nurse.

When implementing the tele-ICU:

- Include ICU clinicians in an early stage in the design and implementation of the tele-ICU.
- Build support for tele-ICU coverage before roll-out.
- Designate an ICU champion.
- If possible, have personnel of the tele-ICU and the ICUs that are to be monitored meet each other. Face-to-face contact reduces many of the barriers that we have found in this study.
- Install 2-way (instead of 1-way) cameras.

After having implemented the tele-ICU:

- If possible, continue to organize meetings in which tele-ICU personnel and ICU personnel can meet. Face-to-face contact reduces many of the barriers that we have found in this study.
- If possible, make a visit to the tele-ICU as part of the educational program for physicians and nurses. Often a visit to the tele-ICU results in a better understanding of what the tele-ICU exactly does (and what it does not do).
- Evidently, tele-ICU personnel would be benefit greatly from standardization in the ICUs that they monitor. However, in many (but not all!) cases tele-ICUs monitor ICUs in separate health systems that use different technology (eg, electronic health records, smart pumps, etc) and processes, which makes a standardized approach very difficult. However, within health care organizations that have several hospitals and ICUs, processes and technology can be standardized with often very positive outcomes.[36] And tele-ICU implementation itself often has some standardization of care as a result.[35]
- Some of the procedures with regard to communication with the ICUs that are monitored can be standardized. This measure creates clearer expectations about responsibilities of the personnel in the ICU and in the tele-ICU.
- Another form of standardization can be achieved by designing policies and procedures for the use of the in-room cameras, speakers, and microphones.[37] The use of this technology often results in the feeling that "Big Brother is watching me" in ICU rooms.
- Hiring tele-ICU nurses who have worked or a still working part time in the ICUs that are monitored does improve the relationship between nurses in the tele-ICU and ICU and increases trust and satisfaction.[8]
- Since 2011, tele-ICU nursing is recognized as a professional specialty and nurses working in the tele-ICU can get a CCRN-E certification.[38] Being a tele-ICU nurse indeed requires specific skills and knowledge to be able to provide care at a distance. Recognizing the difficulties that virtual teamwork can generate, such as having to cope with a large variety of ICU characteristics and the lack of familiarity with the ICU context, but trying to establish relationships and trust with the nurses in the ICUs requires effort from tele-ICU nurses. They should be made aware of these (potential) problems and trained in how to cope with the problems of virtual teams.

REFERENCES

1. Angus DC, Linde-Zwirble WT, Sirio CA, et al. The effect of managed care on ICU length of stay: implications for Medicare. JAMA 1996;276(13):1075–82.
2. Mukhopadhyay A, Tai BC, See KC, et al. Risk factors for hospital and long-term mortality of critically ill elderly patients admitted to an intensive care unit. Biomed Res Int 2014;2014:960575.
3. Breslow MJ. Remote ICU care programs: current status. J Crit Care 2007;22(1): 66–76.
4. Juraschek SP, Zhang X, Ranganathan V, et al. United States registered nurse workforce report card and shortage forecast. Am J Med Qual 2012;27(3):241–9.
5. Bureau of Labor Statistics (BLS). Table 6: the 30 occupations with the largest projected employment growth, 2014-24. Economic News Release 2016. Available at: http://www.bls.gov/news.release/ecopro.t06.htm. Accessed February 2017.
6. Allen L. The nursing shortage continues as faculty shortage grows. Nurs Econ 2008;26(1):35–40.

7. Mullen-Fortino M, DiMartino J, Entrikin L, et al. Bedside nurses' perceptions of intensive care unit telemedicine. Am J Crit Care 2012;21(1):24–32.
8. Hoonakker PLT, Pecanac KE, Brown RL, et al. Virtual collaboration, satisfaction and trust between nurses in the tele-ICU and ICUs: results of a multi-level analysis. J Crit Care 2017;37:224–9.
9. Lilly CM, Thomas EJ. Tele-ICU: experience to date. J Intensive Care Med 2009; 25(1):16–22.
10. Stafford TB, Myers MA, Young A, et al. Working in an eICU unit: life in the box. Crit Care Nurs Clin North Am 2008;20(4):441–50.
11. Tang Z, Weavind L, Mazabob J, et al. Workflow in intensive care unit remote monitoring: a time-and-motion study. Crit Care Med 2007;35(9):2057–63.
12. Hoonakker PLT, Khunlertkit A, Mcguire K, et al. A day in life of a tele-Intensive Care Unit nurse. In: Albolino S, Bagnara S, Bellandi T, et al, editors. Healthcare systems ergonomics and patient safety 2011. Leiden (The Netherlands): CRC Press; 2011. p. 43–6.
13. Nielsen M, Saracino J. Telemedicine in the intensive care unit. Crit Care Nurs Clin North Am 2012;24(3):491–500.
14. Khunlertkit A, Carayon P. Contributions of tele–intensive care unit (Tele-ICU) technology to quality of care and patient safety. J Crit Care 2013;28(3):315.e1-12.
15. Anders S, Patterson ES, Woods DD, et al. Projecting trajectories for a new technology based on cognitive task analysis and archetypal patterns: the electronic ICU. 8th Annual Naturalist Decision Making Conference. Asilomar, CA, June 4–6, 2007.
16. Zawada ETJ, Herr P, Larson D, et al. Impact of an intensive care unit telemedicine program on a rural health care system. Postgrad Med 2009;121(3):160–70.
17. Ries M. Tele-ICU: a new paradigm in critical care. Int Anesthesiol Clin 2009;47(1): 153–70.
18. Thomas EJ, Chu-Weininger MYL, Lucke J, et al. The impact of a tele-ICU provider attitudes about teamwork and safety climate. Crit Care Med 2007;35:A145.
19. Breslow MJ, Rosenfeld BA, Doerfler M, et al. Effect of a multiple-site intensive care unit telemedicine program on clinical and economic outcomes: an alternative paradigm for intensivist staffing. Crit Care Med 2004;32(1):31–8.
20. Willmitch B, Golembeski S, Kim SS, et al. Clinical outcomes after telemedicine intensive care unit implementation. Crit Care Med 2012;40(2):450–4.
21. Chen J, Sun D, Yang W, et al. Clinical and economic outcomes of telemedicine programs in the intensive care unit: a systematic review and meta-analysis. J Intensive Care Med 2017. [EPub ahead of print].
22. Rosenfeld BA, Dorman T, Breslow MJ, et al. Intensive care unit telemedicine: alternate paradigm for providing continuous intensivist care. Crit Care Med 2000;28(12):3925–31.
23. Coustasse A, Deslich S, Bailey D, et al. A business case for tele-intensive care units. Perm J 2014;18(4):76–84.
24. Wilcox ME, Adhikari NK. The effect of telemedicine in critically ill patients: systematic review and meta-analysis. Crit Care 2012;16(4):R127.
25. Young LB, Chan PS, Lu X, et al. Impact of telemedicine intensive care unit coverage on patient outcomes: a systematic review and meta-analysis. Arch Intern Med 2011;171(6):498–506.
26. Kumar S, Merchant S, Reynolds R. Tele-ICU: efficacy and cost-effectiveness of remotely managing critical care. Perspect Health Inf Manag 2013;10:1f.

27. Thomas EJ, Lucke J, Wueste L, et al. Association of telemedicine for remote monitoring of intensive care patients with mortality, complications, and length of stay. JAMA 2009;302(24):2671-8.
28. Morrison JL, Cai Q, Davis N, et al. Clinical and economic outcomes of the electronic intensive care unit: results from two community hospitals. Crit Care Med 2010;38(1):2-8.
29. Cummings J, Krsek C, Vermoch K, et al. Intensive care unit telemedicine: review and consensus recommendations. Am J Med Qual 2007;22(4):239-50.
30. Zuiderent T, Winthereik BR, Berg M. Talking about distributed communication and medicine: on bringing together remote and local actors. Hum Comput Interact 2003;18(1-2):171-80.
31. Young LB, Chan PS, Cram P. Staff acceptance of tele-ICU coverage: a systematic review. Chest 2011;139(2):279-88.
32. Hoonakker PLT, Carayon P, Khunlertkit A, et al. Case study research: an example from the tele-ICU. In: Goebel M, Christie CJ, Zschernack S, et al, editors. Organizational design and management (ODAM), vol. X. Grahamstown (South Africa): IEA Press; 2011. p. 121-7.
33. Yin RK. Case study research: design and methods. Newbury Park (CA): Sage; 1984.
34. Hoonakker PLT, Carayon P, McGuire K, et al. Motivation and job satisfaction of tele-ICU nurses. J Crit Care 2013;28(3):315.e13-21.
35. Goedken CC, Moeckli J, Cram PM, et al. Introduction of tele-ICU in rural hospitals: changing organisational culture to harness benefits. Intensive Crit Care Nurs 2017;40:51-6.
36. Irwin RS, Flaherty HM, French CT, et al. Interdisciplinary collaboration: the slogan that must be achieved for models of delivering critical care to be successful. Chest 2012;142(6):1611-9.
37. Shahpori R, Hebert M, Kushniruk A, et al. Telemedicine in the intensive care unit environment—a survey of the attitudes and perspectives of critical care clinicians. J Crit Care 2011;26(3):328.e9-15.
38. Goran SF. A new view: tele-intensive care unit competencies. Crit Care Nurse 2011;31(5):17-29.

Advancing Continuous Predictive Analytics Monitoring

Moving from Implementation to Clinical Action in a Learning Health System

Jessica Keim-Malpass, PhD, RN[a,b,*],
Rebecca R. Kitzmiller, PhD, MHR, RN, BC[c],
Angela Skeeles-Worley, MEd[d], Curt Lindberg, DMan[e],
Matthew T. Clark, PhD[f,1], Robert Tai, EdD[d],
James Forrest Calland, MD[b], Kevin Sullivan, PhD[g],
J. Randall Moorman, MD[b,f], Ruth A. Anderson, PhD, RN[c]

KEYWORDS

- Predictive analytics monitoring • Implementation science
- Stakeholder driven design • Learning health system • Streaming design

---

Disclosure Statement: J. Keim-Malpass was supported through a grant from the University of Virginia Translational Health Research Institute of Virginia (THRIV) Scholars award. R. Kitzmiller was supported by the National Center for Translational Sciences and National Institutes of Health (NIH) through grant KL2TR001109. The content is solely the responsibility of the authors and does not necessarily represent official views of the NIH. C. Lindberg, R. Anderson, and R. Kitzmiller are supported by MITRE funding agreements 19140 and 11348 (accelerating staff engagement in predictive monitoring development, implementation, and use). The MITRE Corporation operates the Centers for Medicare & Medicaid Services (CMS) Alliance to Modernize Healthcare (CAMH), a federally funded research and development center dedicated to strengthening the nation's health care system. The MITRE Corporation operates CAMH in partnership with the CMS and the Department of Health and Human Services.
Conflicts of Interest: Drs J.R. Moorman and M.T. Clark have equity in, and are officers of, the Advanced Medical Predictive Devices, Diagnostics, and Displays in Charlottesville, VA, USA (AMP3D). Dr M.T Clark is employed by AMP3D.
[a] Department of Acute and Specialty Care, School of Nursing, University of Virginia, PO Box 800782, Charlottesville, VA 22908, USA; [b] Department of Medicine, School of Medicine, University of Virginia, 1215 Lee Street, Charlottesville, VA 22908, USA; [c] School of Nursing, University of North Carolina, Carrington Hall, South Columbia Street, Chapel Hill, NC 27599, USA; [d] School of Education, University of Virginia, 405 Emmet Street South, Charlottesville, VA 22903, USA; [e] Billings Clinic, 801 North 29th Street, Billings, MT 59101, USA; [f] Advanced Medical Predictive Devices, Diagnostics, Displays, Charlottesville, VA 22903, USA; [g] Department of Computer Science, School of Engineering, University of Virginia, Engineer's Way, Charlottesville, VA 22903, USA
[1] 1215 Lee Street, Charlottesville, VA 22908.
* Corresponding author. University of Virginia School of Nursing, PO Box 800782, Charlottesville, VA 22908.
E-mail address: Jlk2t@virginia.edu

Crit Care Nurs Clin N Am 30 (2018) 273–287
https://doi.org/10.1016/j.cnc.2018.02.009
0899-5885/18/© 2018 Elsevier Inc. All rights reserved.

KEY POINTS

- Continuous predictive analytics monitoring synthesizes data from a variety of inputs into a risk estimate that clinicians can observe in a streaming environment.
- For continuous predictive analytics monitoring to be useful, clinicians must engage with the data in a way that makes sense for their clinical workflow in the context of a learning health system (LHS).
- Clinicians described the processes needed to move to clinical action through the following themes: (1) understand the science behind the algorithm, (2) trust the data inputs, (3) integrate with the electronic medical record, and (4) optimize clinical pathways.
- Larger prospective studies are needed to evaluate the relationship between continuous predictive analytics monitoring and clinical action from the lens of LHS and implementation science perspectives.

INTRODUCTION

Intensive care unit (ICU) patients are at the highest level of acuity where they are vulnerable to potentially catastrophic clinical events or complications during the course of their stay.[1] The financial, societal, and human burdens of intensive care are growing[2] and there has been a steady increase in the amount of data inputs received from patients in the ICU. In the ICU, point-of-care clinicians monitor a diverse array of data inputs to detect early signs of impending clinical demise or improvement.[3] Most information gained from unprocessed cardiorespiratory monitoring (multilead electrocardiogram [ECG], pulse waveform, heart rate, respiratory rate, oxygen saturation) is neither fully used nor stored for later analysis.[4] Continuous predictive analytics monitoring synthesizes data from a variety of inputs into a risk estimate that clinicians can observe in a streaming environment.[4,5] The potential applications for streaming continuous predictive analytics monitoring displays in ICU care settings are extensive.[6]

Continuous predictive analytics monitoring was born in the neonatal ICU (NICU).[5,7–13] In the neonatal setting, investigators found abnormal heart rate characteristics (HRCs) in the hours preceding a clinical diagnosis of sepsis.[5] These HRCs were not obvious in vital sign trends, even to experienced clinicians. Methods were developed and refined to characterize, process, and synthesize data inputs. Computational techniques synthesized these data inputs into a model that produced an estimation of risk, which led to the streaming output of characteristics called the HRCs index (**Fig. 1**).[8,13–15] A large, multicenter randomized controlled trial studied the impact of HRC monitoring on patient outcomes and determined a reduction in mortality among very low birth weight infants who were monitored using the HRC index.[8,14] Patients in the HRC monitoring arm received antibiotics for a longer duration of time and clinicians were able to detect preclinical signs of septicemia hours before overt clinical symptoms.[8,14]

The application of continuous predictive analytics monitoring was then extended to critically ill adults.[3,10,11] The first phase necessitated detection of physiologic signatures of illness (prodromes). Emergent intubation and hemorrhage were chosen as the initial clinical outcomes to demonstrate proof of concept and model validation.[3,10,11] The validated algorithms for early detection of subacute and potentially catastrophic illness were then displayed through a continuous streaming environment, called continuous monitoring of event trajectory (CoMET®) (**Fig. 2**). CoMET®

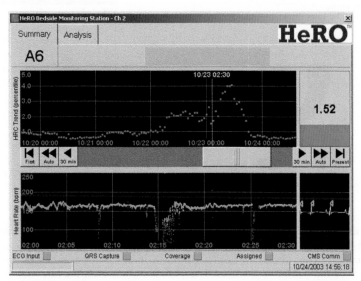

Fig. 1. Bedside implementation of the Heart Rate Observer (HeRO) continuous predictive monitoring. The monitor detects various HRCs and transient decelerations that have been shown to accurately depict septicemia in neonates.[8,14] The HeRO model score of 1.52 represents an odds ratio of risk (ie, a score of 2 would represent a 2-fold risk of the neonate becoming septic). (*Courtesy of* Medical Predictive Science Corporation, Charlottesville, VA.)

has been on display in a surgical trauma burn ICU at an academic medical center since 2015.

For continuous predictive analytics monitoring to be useful, point-of-care clinicians must engage with the data in a way that makes sense for their clinical workflow in the context of a learning health system (LHS). The Institute of Medicine has defined an LHS as, "a vision of an integrated health system in which progress in science, informatics, and care culture align to generate new knowledge as an ongoing natural by-product of the care experience, and seamlessly refines and delivers best practices for continuous improvement in health and healthcare."[16] Initiation of continuous predictive analytics monitoring in an ICU setting represents an opportunity for iterative evaluation and implementation perspectives that align with an LHS approach.[17]

Continuous predictive analytics monitoring relies on the central premise that the technology and computational models will detect early signs of physiologic adverse events, such as cardiorespiratory instability.[18] To affect health outcomes, these technologies must move from active surveillance of physiologic states, such as cardiorespiratory instability, to enhanced clinician-based assessment and clinical action.[18] The necessary processes needed to move from continuous predictive analytics monitoring surveillance to clinical action in an LHS have not been well-described in the scientific literature.[19–21] Therefore, the purpose of this study was to describe the processes needed to evoke clinical action after initiation of continuous predictive analytics monitoring, or CoMET®, in an LHS. Specifically, the authors sought perceptions from point-of-care clinicians as a part of the overall iterative implementation, evaluation, and optimization of this technology in an ICU setting.

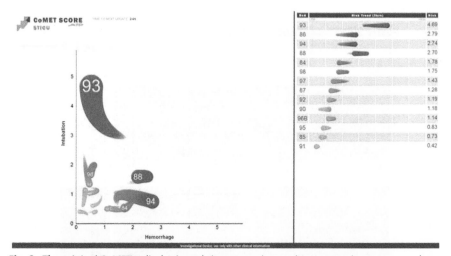

Fig. 2. The original CoMET® display in real-time streaming environment as it appears on a large screen monitor in a unit (dates have been removed). On the left, each patient is represented by a CoMET® with bed number in the head. The x-axis and y-axis show the risk, with respect to average, of emergency intubation or bleeding leading to large transfusion, respectively. Units are increased by fold, so a patient with intubation risk of 1 has average risk for intubation, a patient at 2 has twice the average risk, and so on. The head of the CoMET® represents the current hour, and the tail is 3 hours long. For example, the patient in bed 93 is 5-fold the risk of emergent intubation, up from 3-fold risk 3 hours ago. The right side shows a linearized version of the left plot in which the values are the distance from the origin (coordinates 0,0 on the x-axis and y-axis). In this view, patients are ordered by decreasing risk. The overall rank score of 4.69 represents the combined risk of the intubation and hemorrhage models using the following formula: square root (intubation2 + hemorrhage2). (© 2018 AMP3D Inc.; Charlottesville, VA, USA; with permission. All rights reserved.)

METHODS
Study Design and Sample

This study used a longitudinal qualitative descriptive design using both focus group and individual interviews collected from an academic surgical trauma ICU in central Virginia.[22,23] Participants were recruited through a convenience sampling strategy that included any point-of-care clinician (registered nurse [RN], respiratory therapist, nurse practitioner, attending physician) who worked in the unit and were exposed to CoMET® display monitoring for any period of time. There were no exclusion criteria.

This study included data from 5 focus groups and 14 individual interviews. Invitations to participate were sent through email. Five focus groups were conducted over the course of a year that were audio recorded and included in this analysis. Four of the focus groups had mixed point-of-care clinicians (RN, respiratory therapies, nurse practitioner, or attending physician) and 1 focus group included nurse practitioners and attending physicians. Each focus group ranged from 4 to 6 participants per session and several focus groups included educational content delivered along with semistructured questions to which participants responded. Following the second focus group, feedback was provided to the CoMET® developers and the monitoring platform and visual display were modified. In addition, 7 RNs participated in 2 qualitative individual interviews each, which were conducted about 9 months apart from each other. Observations of unit activity and inpatient rounds were conducted during the study period for context, but were not included as data in this present analysis. Institutional review board approval was obtained before study initiation.

Data Collection and Analysis

Data collection occurred from September 2015 through November 2016. **Table 1** shows relevant timeline associated with data collection. Focus group and individual interviews were conducted using a semistructured interview guide. Questions focused on perceptions of the CoMET® display and use in routine clinical practice. The discussions were audio recorded and transcribed verbatim. Transcripts were then uploaded into a qualitative software management application, Dedoose [Sociocultural Research Consultants (SCRC)].[24] Analytical field notes and observation notes were maintained throughout the data collection time period and were read for context but were not a part of the final data analysis. Data from the 14 individual interviews (n = 7 RNs) and 5 focus groups (n = 26) were included in the final qualitative analysis.

The analytical frame was guided by an open coding strategy applied to the entire data set, followed by an inductive theme development using thematic analysis.[22,23] The text data were analyzed by (1) immersion in the data (ie, reading the transcripts several times for full context), (2) a line-by-line analysis and data reduction in which inductive codes were derived, (3) developing a codebook with newly created code and derived meaning during the coding process, (4) codes were grouped together to form tentative categories and eventual themes.[25] Trustworthiness was addressed in several ways: aspects of the study design were open for review to members of the research team, reflection on prior assumptions and beliefs about the topics discussed, keeping an audit log for analytical decisions, and iterative review of the codes and eventual themes.[26]

RESULTS

Demographic characteristics of the sample were not maintained to protect anonymity because all clinicians were recruited from the same ICU. Several themes and subthemes emerged from the data that described the necessary process to move predictive analytics monitoring from implementation to clinical action. These included

1. Understand the science behind the algorithm (subthemes: first-to-test or lacks standard evidence, and moving to alarm)
2. Trust the data inputs (subtheme: noise).
3. Integrate with the electronic medical record (EMR) (subtheme: treat as vital sign).
4. Optimize clinical pathways (subthemes: reactive to proactive and model refinement).

Sample qualitative exemplars from each theme can be found in **Boxes 1–4**.

Table 1	
Interview structures and Continuous Monitoring of Event Trajectories display timeline	
Time	**Event**
June 2015	CoMET® display monitor mounted in central work station
September 2015	Point-of-care clinician focus group 1
October 2015	Nurse practitioner or attending physician focus group 2
November 2015	Individual interview #1 complete
February 2016	New display features go live based on early focus group feedback
April 2016	Point-of-care clinician focus group 3
December 2016	2 monitors added to front and rear of ICU Individual interview #2 complete

Box 1

Qualitative exemplars of the theme of understanding the science behind the algorithm, and the subthemes of first-to-test or lacks standard evidence, and moving to alarm

It's a bit of a mystery what all those things are, that are being … that are in your algorithm to create that CoMET®. And so it's a mysterious black box (FG1)

[O]ne of my biggest problems was I'd look at it, and then I wouldn't really know what I was actually looking at. There was no handbook to go to. (FG1)

… just being able to see the transparency of what are we looking at. I know that we're talking about—well, we're looking at the vitals, okay. What else are we talking about that's behind this? And then how is it actually presenting back to us? (FG1)

I'm a curious person. I would like to know … for instance what data is going in [to the algorithm], how quickly it's computed, and how delayed is the CoMET® score. What weighs more in this, in the math, I mean, is your oxygen saturation more important than your respiratory rate?, I would like to know that.[6]

For me all I see is two axes and one is hemorrhage and one is intubation. I don't know what data it uses or how frequently it's refreshed or how minute to minute accurate it is.[6]

And just understanding the variables that it takes in and why some outliers can really affect what the CoMET® is doing which I think probably goes back into why … it's not my go to source for information on my patients. (FG2)

[X] told me there was a very big mathematical equation that she didn't even understand, that was coming into play … that weighted certain attributes there. So … I'd love to know how that works, but I know that I wouldn't necessarily understand all the, how each thing gets weighted, … But yes, I would like to … I would like to know more about all of it really.[3]

Nobody really knows what it is and how to access it. I tried to look it up today on the internet. I couldn't find anything about it. I found the company name, but I couldn't find anything about it. (FG1)

You know it seems like when stuff makes it to the bedside it's gone through more rigorous testing. And I think it's more widely accepted. I mean, usually the evidence supports like, using this device or not using this information because it's more risky to insert the device in the first place.[6]

All our patients are monitored of course so we have this real time instant notification with alarms and buzzers and beeps and whistles that tells us exactly when something is going wrong and our brain is already trained to recognize the specific noises that we hear so I feel like we'd hear a respiratory alarm before we'd look and see our CoMET® sway in a certain direction (FG2)

Note: Number corresponds to participant number.
Abbreviation: FG, focus group.

Understand the Science Behind the Algorithm

To fully integrate predictive analytics monitoring capabilities in routine clinical practice, it is necessary for point-of-care clinicians to understand the science behind the algorithm. As 1 clinician described, "I'm a curious person. I would like to know … for instance what is going in [to the algorithm], how quickly it's computed, and how delayed is the CoMET® score. What weighs more in this, in the math, I mean, is your oxygen saturation more important than the respiratory rate? I would like to know that." (Participant #6)

Participants stated that ICU clinicians are so used to understanding how physiologic parameters are calculated that it can be challenging when the calculations underlying the predictive analytics monitoring algorithm are not known. Similarly, it can be frustrating when point-of-care clinicians cannot access data regarding thresholds or

---

Box 2
Qualitative exemplars of the theme trust the data and the subtheme noise

Sometimes I will see that it's different [meaning the CoMET® score and the general assessment of the patient]. Lots of times, honestly, it's because the data is wrong that's going into the CoMET® score. The data, for some reason, said the pressures were low because the A-line was kinked. Or the respirations were zero when it was not, that kind of thing. The CoMET® is soaring, but [the patient] is actually okay. Then sometimes they are real. They do kind of correlate with it. Sometimes I'll look at a patient and not really be able to put words to what's wrong. Then their CoMET® is higher, wider, whatever.[14]

It is difficult I think sometimes in the ICU to really see if there's been trends because they have been in the hospital for so long or they have blood pressure medications they are on, so with that playing in to account for their heart rate and their blood pressure depending then it is not really giving us an accurate CoMET® score.[13]

I think there is some reservation about the data that's incorporated, because I feel like it's reliant upon us as nurses to validate vital signs and information appropriately. Sometimes it's easy to validate information that could accidently be incorrect. We have somebody that's on a ventilator ... from the vent, we get their respiratory rate. However, we had leads on their chest that also has a respiratory rate, and maybe those leads aren't placed appropriately and so we're getting an inflated value of, I don't know, maybe 50. [W]e're reliant on what we know the vent's programmed to do. When we're validating our vital signs, it's can be really easy to click here and validate, versus looking at it intentionally and focused on making sure that it's accurate.[12]

We can choose not to validate that reading [the vital sign]. If we're not careful, almost like alarm fatigue. If you're not careful, you can just automatically validate it not realizing—you know what I mean? Certain things like that can happen and maybe throw off your CoMET® score.[7]

[You'll see] someone's CoMET® score is sky-high, and yet that patient's already intubated, and you're like, "Oh, the respiration rate isn't accurate.[5]

I think that it [the CoMET® model] has a lot of potential. I think the part that's challenging is making sure that the information that they are utilizing to make the calculation is accurate. I think that's always going to be a struggle. I just don't think that—I don't know how you would ever make that accurate, because you can have your leads on, which is measuring an EKG [sic] rhythm, and also a respiration rate that's not accurate. The reason we know an accurate respiration rate is because we can go and look at our ventilator.[5]

I can see where the information could be really good, because you can see if a patient was becoming febrile, they're going become tachycardic. It's just figuring out the accuracy of the information that they're using.[5]

There's sometimes I see it's my patient and I'm like why is their CoMET® score so high? My first instinct is to make sure like the leads are reading accurately (FG2)

Note: Number corresponds to participant number.
Abbreviation: FG, focus group.

---

cutoffs. Usually when monitoring or clinical decision support devices are deployed at the bedside, they have been rigorously tested through randomized clinical trials and have information on interpretation readily accessible through peer-reviewed manuscripts. Another clinician articulated the challenges associated with being the first to test the monitoring device in the following statement: "[O]ne of my biggest problems was I'd look at it, and then I wouldn't really know what I was looking at. There was no handbook to go to." (Focus group 1)

Because alarms are so ubiquitous with ICU care delivery, several participants noted that it was challenging to keep up with the CoMET® display because there was not an

---

Box 3
Qualitative exemplars of the theme integrate with electronic medical record and the subtheme treat as vital sign

We open up this document or program for charting. We open up another program for label printing for our blood-work. Then it's a third thing to open up CoMET®. I think that's probably the main barrier. Is that we're all on one screen, and we're opening—there's just multiple programs to open up.[11]

If I want to see their last 24 hours over a timeframe I always pull it up on the computer. But I definitely don't like leave it on the background of the computer all the time. Since we recently just got badge scanners that pretty much allow us to stay logged in in the background I think it might be simpler to pull it up on the screen and have it just open up when we open the computer but the way we logged in and out before you constantly would have to click on it and log back into it.[13]

There's been discussion of trying to incorporate the CoMET® score into our vital signs, so it would be something we were validating every hour as well as into the daily rounds that happen in the morning with the LIPs [licensed independent provider] the nurse, the respiratory therapist and the charge nurse, so it would be incorporated into that daily routine to see if more discussion of it consistently at a specific time it would get more people to pay attention to it throughout the day.[13]

If we were able to incorporate our CoMET® score within our vital signs and something that is, right within Epic would be huge.[9]

I feel maybe if that was CoMET®—if it just got pulled over into our vitals or something like that, it wouldn't just get forgotten about.[8]

I think linking it to Epic would be really helpful because every hour we're required to go in and validate our vital signs so and naturally of course we're required to look like what's their heart rate, what's their blood pressure and that sort of thing and so if we could have just a row in Epic that says their CoMET® score just went from 2, if it was on a scale of twenty, two to twenty or something like that then that would be something to pay attention to. (FG2)

I don't think that there's a way right now to have it pulled in. Our monitors pull in our data, and then we validate that every hour. I don't think that the CoMET® score is attached, so to speak, to Epic. Our last group meeting, we were talking about different ways to try to develop that because we can tailor Epic to do that kind of thing. If it can show up on our desktop, we're trying to find a way to make it show up in Epic. Then we can validate that like we would another vital sign.[10]

I don't think it would be [a big deal to document as a vital sign in the EMR] ... I'm sure some people are always going to complain and say ... "one more thing to document" you know?[3]

Note: Number corresponds to participant number.
Abbreviation: FG, focus group.

---

alarm, trigger, or threshold associated with the number. The desire for a cut-off or threshold to initiate clinical action represented a prominent subtheme. As stated, "All our patients are monitored of course so we have this real time instant notification with alarms and buzzers and beeps and whistles that tells us exactly when something is going wrong and our brain is already trained to recognize the specific noises that we hear so I feel like we'd hear a respiratory alarm before we'd look and see our CoMET® sway in a certain direction." (Focus group 2)

Moving to an alarm-based system represents a necessary process that incorporates understanding the science in a way that refines continuous predictive analytical scores into appropriate clinical thresholds to respond to. The subtheme of moving to alarm was articulated by several clinicians as a step necessary to later evoke a clinical action.

Box 4
Qualitative exemplars of the theme optimize clinical pathways and the subthemes reactive to proactive and model refinement

That's not our culture yet, to really be referencing the CoMET® score as a part of our report, or as a part of our discussion with one another. It's really just something that we'll look at, and see where our patients fall. I don't know if we're really using it to create interventions yet.[1]

Being able to do something with CoMET® scores, where it's saying, based on these changes this might be what ... this might be one pathway. (FG1)

Then I looked at the monitor and it was like, "Oh yeah, the heart rates are a little bit higher than when I thought there were. The pressures have started softening a little bit." I think we did another ABG [arterial blood gas] and I sent off a complete—a CBC [complete blood count] to get the make-up of the blood to see if we had a volume issue with the hemoglobin or hematocrit. We did, so we needed to get some volume.[12]

It's not something titratable, right. There's no drug that is, for lowering your CoMET® score. I think that sometimes what we're doing is we're focusing on numbers and specific numbers that we can treat and alter.[8]

The vital signs are something I can take at the bedside and act pretty instantly on. You know. If somebody's blood pressure is high and I need to bring it down I can see it, I can act on it, I can see it's result instantly. Heart rate, for instance, if ... if I know the source then ... you know ... I'm at the bedside treating the source of the high heart rate, you know, temperature. It's ... I guess it's different [CoMET®] in the sense of the immediacy that I can interpret, act, and then also reassess the data.[6]

And then in turn having that active role for the bedside clinician, the LIP [licensed independent provider] will then foster buy-in, and it makes it part of our workflow and makes us attuned to the number. This is the scenario. This is what we were seeing beforehand. This is what you did. This is what we saw afterward. This is the effect that you all had." (FG 2)

[We need to] kind of change our culture from the reactive to a proactive environment.[1]

It would be useful if we were able to take into account interventions that are happening. For example, if a patient already is on a ventilator, their risk for intubation shouldn't necessarily be high. It kind of distorts the people's value that they place in it, because then they see this person who has the largest CoMET® on the board. They're already intubated. Really, looking at that would be nice if they could include interventions. There's almost no way that there would be a streamlined, easy process for that to be implemented in something like this. That would be nice, but would be more so of a dream, I think, than a reality.[1]

Even just like basic having a hemoglobin and hematocrit included into it at least then we'd see are they losing blood, do they need something else, do they need more blood. It would show that and giving the blood products sure we are going to be giving them the volume but their blood pressure would have to improve and then their cardiovascular instability would go down if we were doing that.[13]

The main thing is we're all very interested in having lab values incorporated in it [CoMET®], especially for their risk of hemorrhage, or even if they're able to use ABGs [arterial blood gases] to be looking at their Po_2 [partial pressure of oxygen] and their SATs [saturations] as well on their blood gasses, instead of just looking at what their SATs are on the pulse ox. Because sometimes even the vital signs that are coming up on our monitor aren't necessarily accurate to the patient. Depending on who it is and their blood focus in general.[1]

Note: Number corresponds to participant number.
Abbreviation: FG, focus group.

Trust the Data Inputs

To move across the continuum from implementation of continuous predictive analytics to a resulting clinical action based on a model score, clinicians also articulated they need to trust the data inputs that support the predictive model. Because the clinicians understood that the predictive model was calculated based on the vital sign data they entered and validated in the EMR, the concept of accurate data validation was central to many of the interviews, as described by the following 2 statements.

First statement: "I think there is some reservation about the data that's incorporated, because I feel like it's reliant upon us as nurses to validate vital signs and information appropriately. Sometimes it's easy to validate information that could accidently be incorrect. We have somebody that's on a ventilator … from the vent, we get their respiratory rate. However, we had leads on their chest that also has a respiratory rate, and maybe those leads aren't placed appropriately and so we're getting an inflated value of, I don't know, maybe 50. [W]e're reliant on what we know the vent's programmed to do. When we're validating our vital signs, it's can be really easy to click here and validate, versus looking at it intentionally and focused on making sure that it's accurate." (Participant #12)

Second statement: "We can choose not to validate that reading [the vital sign that is, inaccurate]. If we're not careful, almost like alarm fatigue, you can just automatically validate it not realizing—you know what I mean? Certain things like that can happen and maybe throw off your CoMET® score." (Participant #7)

A subtheme that was critical to this discourse was the noise that skews the predictive model, due to incorrect data inputs. A description of noise is represented by the following excerpt: "I think that it [the CoMET® model] has a lot of potential. I think the part that's challenging is making sure that the information that they are utilizing to make the calculation is accurate. I think that's always going to be a struggle. I just don't think that—I don't know how you would ever make that accurate, because you can have your leads on, which is measuring an EKG [sic] rhythm, and also a respiration rate that's not accurate. The reason we know an accurate respiration rate is because we can go and look at our ventilator." (Participant #5)

The topic of incorrect respiratory leads as a potential problem affecting the model was a pervasive barrier that was noted in almost all of the interviews. It was clear that point-of-care clinicians must trust the data inputs that build the predictive model before fully adopting any subsequent action into routine practice.

Integrate with the Electronic Medical Record

Participants uniformly suggested that integration within the EMR (ie, Epic [Epic Systems, Corporated]) would be a critical component of successful adoption of CoMET®. Some participants noted that it would be advantageous to be able to pull in the data points directly into the flowsheets, just as the EMR is able to do with other vital sign entries. Clinicians described this interface in the following 2 passages.

First statement: "I don't think that there's a way right now to have it pulled in. Our monitors pull in our data, and then we validate that every hour. I don't think that the CoMET® score is attached, so to speak, to Epic. Our last group meeting, we were talking about different ways to try to develop that because we can tailor Epic to do that kind of thing. If it can show up on our desktop, we're trying to find a way to make it show up in Epic. Then we can validate that like we would another vital sign." (Participant #10)

Second statement: "I think linking it to Epic would be really helpful because every hour we're required to go in and validate our vital signs so and naturally of course we're required to look like what's their heart rate, what's their blood pressure and that sort of thing and so if we could have just a row in Epic that says their CoMET® score just went from two, if it was on a scale of twenty, two to twenty or something like that then that would be something to pay attention to." (Focus group 2)

Related to integration with the EMR is the perception that by doing so clinicians are able to treat the CoMET® score as a vital sign that can be responded to with clinical action. There was strong sentiment that treating CoMET® as a vital sign through integration of the EMR and acknowledgment of the result would lead to more attention to the score as a trend. As stated, "There's been discussion of trying to incorporate the CoMET® score into our vital signs, so it would be something we were validating every hour as well as into the daily rounds that happen in the morning with the LIPs [licensed independent providers], the nurse, the respiratory therapist and the charge nurse, so it would be incorporated into that daily routine to see if more discussion of it consistently at a specific time it would get more people to pay attention to it throughout the day." (Participant #13)

An unintended consequence of integration with the EMR and validation of the CoMET® score as a vital sign could be the increased burden on point-of-care clinicians. Even so, the critical component of acknowledgment and documentation was overwhelmingly described as a necessary component of adoption to move to clinical action.

Optimize Clinical Pathways

Clinicians discussed optimization of clinical pathways as a way of describing how the CoMET® score could be turned into a threshold or alarm that would initiate a specific clinical action. One clinician described that the unit was not at the point of adoption yet in the following statement, "That's not our culture yet, to really be referencing the CoMET® score as a part of our report, or as a part of our discussion with one another. It's really just something that we'll look at, and see where our patients fall. I don't know if we're really using it to create interventions yet." (Participant #1)

Another clinician described how she was able to use a rising CoMET® score as a trigger for subsequent clinical action in the following example: "[After noticing a rising CoMET® score] Then I looked at the monitor and it was like, 'Oh yeah, the heart rates are a little bit higher than when I thought there were. The pressures have started softening a little bit.' I think we did another ABG [arterial blood gas] and I sent off a complete—a CBC [complete blood count] to get the make-up of the blood to see if we had a volume issue with the hemoglobin or hematocrit. We did, so we needed to get some volume." (Participant #12)

Because the CoMET® model is predicting an adverse event in the future, many noted that a rising CoMET® score may evoke a different sense of clinical immediacy than a rising heart rate. A clinician described that the clinical response to CoMET® would have to change from a reactive to proactive environment to elicit appropriate action. Several clinicians perceived that allowing for further model refinement could help optimize the clinical response, as described in the following statement: "The main thing is we're all very interested in having lab values incorporated in it [CoMET®], especially for their risk of hemorrhage, or even if they're able to use ABGs [arterial blood gases] to be looking at their Po_2 [partial pressure of oxygen] and their SATs [saturations] as well on their blood gasses, instead of just looking at what their SATs are on the pulse ox[imeter]. Because sometimes even the vital signs that are coming up on our monitor aren't necessarily accurate to the patient. Depending on who it is and their blood focus in general." (Participant #1)

None of the point-of-care clinicians expressed that CoMET® was at the point of adoption at which it was amenable to a clinical protocol (ie, if CoMET® reaches X, then do Y, Z); however, several of the participants were interested in refining certain models and determining appropriate CoMET® threshold limits that could elicit specific clinical actions.

Feedback from the first 2 focus groups was used by the CoMET® developers to revise the display (**Fig. 3**). Handbooks for the CoMET® monitor were distributed to the unit to describe the science behind the algorithm (theme 1), define the filtering used by the platform (theme 3), and provide example cases for proactive use of CoMET® (theme 4). Integration with the EMR was added to CoMET® and risk estimates populate the Epic flowsheet hourly (theme 3).

DISCUSSION

There is a gap in the literature of research focused on implementation of continuous predictive analytics monitoring. Even less known about how to optimize the implementation among a clinician user group that is the first to test the modality in practice.

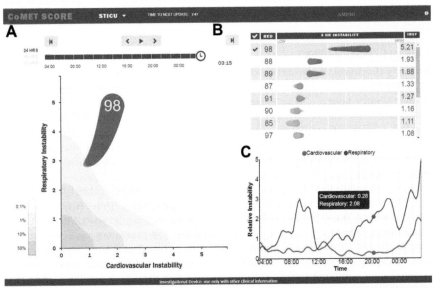

Fig. 3. The CoMET® display with new features based on stakeholder feedback (dates have been removed). On (*B*), the single patient in bed 98 has been selected for closer inspection. Selecting the individual patient brings up (*C*), and all other patients are temporarily removed from (*A*). The axes have been relabeled in terms of system instability. Grayscale contours in the background of (*A*) show percentiles of instability measures, with a legend to the left. The darkest gray represents the 50th percentile, followed by the 10th, and so forth. The current time on the display is 03:15. Play-back tools appear at the top of 3A when the patient is selected, allowing clinicians to review up to 72 hours of monitoring time. Currently, 24 hours is selected and the patient's instability over the preceding 24 hours is shown in the bottom right (*C*) for respiratory (*green*) and cardiovascular (*orange*) systems. Hovering the mouse over the instability lines shows a tooltip with precise values of the instability at that time. As shown in (*B, C*), the respiratory instability at 03:15 is currently 5-fold the average; the tooltip shows that the instability increased greater than 2-fold at 20:00 the previous night, 7 hours earlier. The patient was emergently intubated at 04:45. (© 2018 AMP3D Inc.; with permission. All rights reserved.)

Point-of-care clinicians in this study articulated that understanding these implementation processes in an LHS are critical steps that are needed before any resulting clinical action. The LHS offers a system of care that allows for exploration of systematic approaches to health delivery based on integrated predictive physiologic data used in a complex clinical milieu.[4] For continuous predictive analytics monitoring to be viewed as a means of clinical decision support, clinicians in this study attested that the processes that are necessary for adoption include understanding the science behind the algorithm, trusting the data, integrating with the EMR, and optimizing clinical pathways.

The process of adoption from implementation to clinical action is even more complex among this user group because they were the first to test the visual streaming display. Although the CoMET® algorithms had been tested and validated,[3,10,11] corresponding clinical thresholds and specific clinical actions are still to be developed. Point-of-care clinicians, particularly nurses and respiratory therapists, are used to alarms, vital sign thresholds, triggers, and clinical protocols as a part of their ICU culture of care.[27–30] Their desires to transform CoMET® through the various processes was articulated as a parallel approach in implementation.

The authors' analysis describes the processes needed before evoking clinical action after initiation of continuous predictive analytics monitoring in an LHS in a surgical trauma ICU located in an academic medical center. This analysis prioritizes the perspectives of the point-of-care clinicians actively working in the environment and allows for tailored iteration based on the specific unit culture of the LHS. Nurses have the opportunity to transform care from reactive to proactive and (1) potentially reduce catastrophic events and complications for their patients and (2) use the data to determine stability and promote nursing care that is patient-centered and beneficial to overall clinical outcomes.

Limitations exist in this study that must be addressed. Because clinicians were all recruited from the same ICU in a single academic medical center and a qualitative methodology was used, results may lack generalizability to other care settings. Additionally, there was a heterogeneity of point-of-care clinicians and experience mix in the sample. Even so, there were several advantages in that the perceptions elicited were from multiple stakeholder groups (RNs, respiratory therapy, nurse practitioner, attending physician). Finally, because this study was longitudinal, the authors were able to account for various levels of exposure to the CoMET® display in the analysis. This study suggests that larger prospective studies with quantitative measures are needed to evaluate the relationship between CoMET® display and clinical action from the lens of LHS and implementation science perspectives.

REFERENCES

1. Stockwell DC, Kane-Gill SL. Developing a patient safety surveillance system to identify adverse events in the intensive care unit. Crit Care Med 2010;38(6): S117–25.
2. Adhikari NKJ, Rubenfeld GD. Worldwide demand for critical care. Curr Opin Crit Care 2011;17(6):620–5.
3. Politano AD, Riccio LM, Lake DE, et al. Predicting the need for urgent intubation in a surgical/trauma intensive care unit. Surgery 2013;154(5):1110–6.
4. Celi L. Big data in the intensive care unit. Closing the data loop. Am J Respir Crit Care Med 2013;187(11):1157–60.
5. Lake DE, Fairchild KD, Moorman JR. Complex signals bioinformatics: evaluation of heart rate characteristics monitoring as a novel risk marker for neonatal sepsis. J Clin Monit Comput 2014;28(4):329–39.

6. Wilbanks BA, Langford PA. A review of dashboards for data analytics in nursing. Comput Inform Nurs 2014;32(11):545–9.

7. Moss TJ, Calland JF, Enfield KB, et al. New-onset atrial fibrillation in the critically Ill. Crit Care Med 2017;45(5):790–7.

8. Fairchild K, Schelonka R, Kaufman D, et al. Septicemia mortality reduction in neonates in a heart rate characteristics monitoring trial. Pediatr Res 2013;74(5):570–5.

9. Clark MT, Delos JB, Lake DE, et al. Stochastic modeling of central apnea events in preterm infants. Physiol Meas 2016;37(4):463–84.

10. Moss TJ, Clark MT, Lake DE, et al. Heart rate dynamics preceding hemorrhage in the intensive care unit. J Electrocardiol 2015;48(6):1075–80.

11. Moss TJ, Lake DE, Calland JF, et al. Signatures of subacute potentially catastrophic illness in the ICU: model development and validation. Crit Care Med 2016;44(9):1639–48.

12. Blackburn HN, Clark MT, Moss TJ, et al. External validation in an intermediate unit of a respiratory decompensation model trained in an intensive care unit. Surgery 2017;161(3):760–70.

13. Sullivan BA, McClure C, Hicks J, et al. Early heart rate characteristics predict death and morbidities in preterm infants. J Pediatr 2016;174:57–62.

14. Moorman JR, Carlo WA, Kattwinkel J, et al. Mortality reduction by heart rate characteristic monitoring in very low birth weight neonates: a randomized trial. J Pediatr 2011;159(6):900–7.

15. Fairchild K, Aschner. HeRO monitoring to reduce mortality in NICU patients. Res Rep Neonatol 2012;65.

16. IOM, Aschner JL. Digital infrastructure for the learning health system. In: Grossman C, Powers B, McGinnis J, editors. The Foundation for Continuous Improvement in Health and Health Care. Washington, DC: National Academy of Medicine; 2011. p. 1–311.

17. Liu VX, Morehouse JW, Baker JM, et al. Data that drive: closing the loop in the learning hospital system. J Hosp Med 2016;11(Suppl 1):S11–7.

18. Bose E, Hoffman L, Hravnak M. Monitoring cardiorespiratory instability: current approaches and implications for nursing practice. Intensive Crit Care Nurs 2016;34:73–80.

19. Osheroff JA, Teich JM, Middleton B, et al. A roadmap for national action on clinical decision support. J Am Med Inform Assoc 2007;14(2):141–5.

20. Alam N, Hobbelink EL, van Tienhoven AJ, et al. The impact of the use of the Early Warning Score (EWS) on patient outcomes: a systematic review. Resuscitation 2014;85(5):587–94.

21. Saunders R, Smith MD. The path to continuously learning health care. Vol 29. Washington, DC: National Academy of Medicine; 2013. https://doi.org/10. 17226/13444.

22. Sandelowski M. What's in a name? Qualitative description revisited. Res Nurs Health 2010;33:77–84.

23. Sandelowski M. Focus on research methods whatever happened to qualitative description? Res Nurs Health 2000;23:334–40.

24. SocioCultural Research Consultants L. Dedoose.

25. Cohen MZ, Kahn DL, Steeves RH. Hermeneutic phenomenological research. Thousand Oaks (CA): Sage; 2000. Available at: http://books.google.com/books/about/Hermeneutic_phenomenological_research.html?id=jPlqRic8TXMC. Accessed March 27, 2012.

26. Lincoln Y, Guba E. Naturalistic inquiry. Beverly Hills (CA): Sage Publications; 1985.
27. Gorges M, Markewitz BA, Westenskow DR. Improving alarm performance in the medical intensive care unit using delays and clinical context. Anesth Analg 2009; 108(5):1546–52.
28. Siebig S, Kuhls S, Imhoff M, et al. Intensive care unit alarms—how many do we need?*. Crit Care Med 2010;38(2):451–6.
29. Nelson JE, Curtis JR, Mulkerin C, et al. Choosing and using screening criteria for palliative care consultation in the ICU: a report from the Improving Palliative Care in the ICU (IPAL-ICU) Advisory Board. Crit Care Med 2013;41(10):2318–27.
30. Deindl P, Unterasinger L, Kappler G, et al. Successful implementation of a neonatal pain and sedation protocol at 2 NICUs. Pediatrics 2013;132(1):e211–8.

Telemedicine in the Intensive Care Unit
Improved Access to Care at What Cost?

William J. Binder, PharmD[a], Jennifer L. Cook, MD[a],*,
Nickalaus Gramze, MD[b], Sophia Airhart, MD[c]

KEYWORDS

* Tele-ICU * eICU * Telemedicine * Critical care * Intensive care unit

KEY POINTS

* Telemedicine programs in the intensive care unit (ICU) have demonstrated mortality and length-of-stay benefits within an ICU stay and possibly to an entire hospital stay.
* Variations exist among tele-ICU programs and future investigations should identify individual components essential to patient outcomes.
* Specific populations that may benefit the most from tele-ICU programs have not been identified.
* Despite large initial costs and logistical planning to implement a tele-ICU program, the potential financial benefits and improved outcomes may provide motivation for widespread adoption.

INTRODUCTION

Due to advances in telemedicine, nurses and physicians are able to provide services in real time from remote locations. Telemedicine is used in virtually all specialties, in both hospital and out-of-hospital settings. According to a 2015 report, telemedicine is incorporated in the care of 13% of intensive care unit (ICU) patients in the United States.[1] Geographic challenges and a growing nurse and physician workforce shortage affect patients' access to specialized care. Telemedicine expands the reach of specialized care and removes geographic barriers. Telemedicine was adapted early in the outpatient setting; however, recent technological advances make it possible to observe and treat patients in critical care settings, where rapid and accurate assessment has an immediate impact on life and death.

Disclosure Statement: The authors report no financial disclosures.
[a] University of Arizona College of Medicine, 1501 North Campbell Avenue, Tucson, AZ 85724, USA; [b] Banner University Medical Center Phoenix, 755 East McDowell Road, Phoenix, AZ 85006, USA; [c] University of Arizona College of Medicine, Sarver Heart Center, 1501 North Campbell Avenue, Room 5157-A, PO Box 245046, Tucson, AZ 85718, USA
* Corresponding author.
E-mail address: jencook@shc.arizona.edu

This staffing challenge in America's ICUs is followed by Leapfrog, a well-known patient safety coalition, that reports that in many areas hospitals are unable to meet staffing standards for intensive care specialized nurses and providers (**Box 1**).[2–4] Hospitals are affected by a workforce shortage of intensivists and in smaller (often rural) hospitals, the financial burden of providing full 24-hour services for a small patient census can be prohibitive.[3] This could escalate to a public health crisis, as it is reasonable to expect that with our aging population, the critical care demands will further increase on the already stretched workforce. Telemedicine in the ICU (tele-ICU) may offer a potential solution to address this pressing need.

WHAT IS THE TELEMEDICINE IN THE INTENSIVE CARE UNIT PRACTICE MODEL?

Tele-ICU is defined as "two-way audio-visual patient monitoring systems that link physicians and nurses who specialize in critical care medicine in a command center to care for ICU patients in multiple, distant units."[5] This technology marries audio and visual hardware components with intelligent software programs to detect physiologic changes in a patient's condition. Typically, a status change in the patient's condition would stimulate an automated alert to the centralized command center where specialists then collaborate with local staff to intervene. The specific design of tele-ICU systems varies; however, there are components common to all tele-ICUs (**Box 2**).[5,6] The command center typically employs a complete critical care team, including intensivists, nurses, and support staff. They may be located within the hospital monitoring several ICUs or in some cases are at a remote location monitoring several hospitals. Services may be offered 24 hours a day or just cover after hours when providers are not in the hospital. A customized tele-ICU model can serve as the primary caregiving team or act as an adjunct when a patient becomes unstable.[6] Several interventions are associated with lower patient mortality and length of stay (LOS), and include (1) intensivist case review within 1 hour of ICU admission, (2) frequent collaborative review of data, (3) adherence to ICU best practices, and (4) quicker alert response times (**Table 1**).[7] It has been shown that the option of tele-ICU remote consultation alone is not enough, and that active monitoring with alerts is necessary to affect outcomes.[7,8]

A survey of 170 active tele-ICUs was conducted in 2009.[8] On average, tele-ICU services were provided 16.5 hours a day (range 10–24 hours). Remote critical care teams were composed of providers and nurses at a ratio of roughly 1:3. In some cases, on-site staff included intensive care physicians; however, it was commonly reported that trainee physicians and nonphysician practitioners provided the local care. With protocols that use monitoring software and sufficient staffing to triage, a single intensivist

---

Box 1

Summary of Leapfrog intensive care unit (ICU) physician staffing requests

- $\geq$1 board-certified intensivist managing all patients
- Intensivists present daily in a single ICU for 8 hours in daytime
- Pages returned within 5 minutes ($\geq$95% of the time) when not physically present
- On-site physician or clinical staff within 5 minutes of ICU patients

Data from Castlight Health and The Leapfrog Group. Intensive care unit physician staffing: data by hospital on nationally standardized metrics. Available at: http://www.leapfroggroup.org/sites/default/files/Files/Castlight-Leapfrog-ICU-Physician-Staffing-Report-2016.pdf. Accessed October 10, 2017.

Box 2
Key components of telemedicine ICUs

- Intensivists managing care from remote command center
- Two-way monitoring systems with audio-visual communication
- Alarms for patient status changes
- Management protocols incorporated into monitoring system

Data from New England Healthcare Institute and Massachusetts Technology Collaborative. Critical care, critical choices: the case for tele-ICUs in intensive care. Available at: https://masstech.org/sites/mtc/files/documents/2010 TeleICU Report.pdf. Accessed October 10, 2017.

---

may cover up to 150 patients.[1] This model has potential to provide an answer for centers lacking specialists and may help medicine prepare for upcoming swell in demand.

WHAT EVIDENCE EXISTS REGARDING TELEMEDICINE IN THE INTENSIVE CARE UNIT OUTCOMES?

The challenge to understanding studies reporting outcomes of tele-ICU care is the substantial variation among tele-ICU models, as well as a lack of randomized data. Common outcomes are survival and LOS measured during ICU stay as well as to discharge from the hospital. A significant number of observational reports comparing outcomes before and after tele-ICU integration are available in the literature.[7,9–15]

Three published meta-analyses report aggregate single-center experiences.[16–18] Reduction in ICU mortality and ICU LOS were consistently reported (**Table 2**). In 2011, Young and colleagues[17] reported that although there was improvement in ICU mortality and LOS following tele-ICU implementation, the effect was neutral

---

Table 1
Outcome measures associated with specific interventions

	Outcome Association			
Intervention Type	Hospital Mortality Benefit	ICU Mortality Benefit	Hospital LOS Reduction	ICU LOS Reduction
Intensivist review of the care plan within 1 h of admission	✔	✔	✔	✔
More frequent collaborative review	✔	—	✔	—
Increased adherence to ICU best practices	✔	—	✔	—
Shorter response times to alarms	—	—	—	✔
Interdisciplinary rounds	✔	—	—	—
Institutional ICU committee effectiveness	✔	—	—	—

Abbreviations: ICU, intensive care unit; LOS, length of stay.
Data from Lilly CM, McLaughlin JM, Zhao H, et al. A multicenter study of ICU telemedicine reengineering of adult critical care. Chest 2014;145(3):500–7.

Table 2
Summary of meta-analysis study results

Study	Total Number of Studies	ICU-Specific Findings		In-Hospital Findings	
		Mortality	**LOS**	**Mortality**	**LOS**
Young et al,[17] 2011	13	12 studies OR = 0.80 (95% CI, 0.66–0.97; P = .02)	7 studies 1.26-d mean reduction (95% CI, −2.21 to −0.30; P = .01)	10 studies OR = 0.82 (95% CI, 0.65–1.03; P = .08)	6 studies 0.64-d mean reduction (95% CI, −1.52–0.25; P = .16)
Wilcox & Adhikari,[16] 2012	11	9 studies RR = 0.79 (95% CI, 0.65–0.96; P = .02)	7 studies WMD = −0.62 d (95% CI, −1.21 to −0.04 d; P = .04)	9 studies RR = 0.83 (95% CI, 0.73–0.94; P = .004)	6 studies WMD = −1.26 d (95% CI, −2.49 to −0.03 d; P = .04)
Chen et al,[18] 2017	19	15 studies RR = 0.83 (95% CI, 0.72–0.96; P = .01)	9 studies WMD = −0.63 d (95% CI, −1.09 to −0.17 d; P = .007)	13 studies RR = 0.74 (95% CI, 0.58–0.96; P = .02)	8 studies WMD = −0.27 d (95% CI, −1.14–0.59 d; P = .54)

Abbreviations: CI, confidence interval; ICU, intensive care unit; LOS, length of stay; OR, odds ratio; RR, risk ratio; WMD, weighted-mean difference.
Data from Refs.[16–18]

with regard to mortality or LOS when comparing the in-hospital outcomes defined as entire hospital stay from admission to discharge. A later study published in 2012 reported improvement of in-hospital mortality and LOS, as well as outcomes within the ICU alone.[16] The most recent and largest meta-analysis was published by Chen and colleagues[18] in 2017. This meta-analysis of 19 studies reported decreased ICU and in-hospital mortality, and improved ICU LOS but no difference in total in-hospital LOS.

Although most studies available compare pre–tele-ICU and post–tele-ICU implementation outcomes, 3 notable studies were strengthened by including a comparison group. The first, published by Nassar and colleagues,[14] reported pre-implementation and post-implementation including a nonintervention ICU group as a control. In a risk-adjusted analysis accounting for patient demographics, co-morbid illnesses, primary ICU admission diagnosis, and selected laboratory values, no differences were found in mortality or LOS in the tele-ICUs compared with nonintervention ICUs. A second large study, by Lilly and colleagues,[7] included 19 health care systems and 118,990 patients (107,432 intervention and 11,558 control). All tele-ICUs used the same audio/video hardware and physiologic software; however, the individual unit procedures and protocols were not standardized. Although Nassar and colleagues[14] did not report differences between the intervention and control groups, in this larger cohort Lilly and colleagues[7] reported decreased hospital mortality, decreased ICU mortality, and decreased hospital LOS. Again, lack of standardization in management protocols challenge the ability to critically evaluate outcomes across existing studies. In a final study, Kahn and colleagues[19] reviewed the outcomes of Medicare beneficiaries admitted to 1 of 132 tele-ICU hospitals (compared with 389 control hospitals). In this study, a small, but statistically significant mortality benefit was seen in pooled data; however, the mortality benefit was shown in only 16 individual hospitals. When considered alone, urban hospitals and hospitals with high patient volume demonstrated mortality benefit after adoption of the tele-ICU system.

In addition to overall mortality and LOS outcomes, a 2011 study assessed the effect of a tele-ICU program on the adherence to clinical practice guidelines and occurrence of ICU-related complications.[20] Patients were significantly more likely to receive prophylaxis for stress ulcers and deep vein thrombosis. Adherence to best practice guidelines for cardiovascular protection was significantly greater after tele-ICU monitoring. This improved adherence to best practices with tele-ICU implementation decreased preventable complications such as ventilator-associated pneumonia and catheter-related bloodstream infections.

WHAT BARRIERS EXIST TO WIDESPREAD IMPLEMENTATION?

Implementation of a new tele-ICU program requires installation of audio and video hardware within each patient room, which may require lengthy retrofitting that creates down time in bed utilization. Poor interoperability between the new software and the hospital's native electronic medical record systems was cited as a barrier in a 2007 survey of adopting and nonadopting hospitals.[21] For example, basic vital signs and laboratory data automatically crossed over from the hospital electronic medical record to the tele-ICU program; however, other critical data, such as fluid status, medications, and ventilator settings did not. Although tele-ICU software program may be robust in features, it is limited by the availability of patient data accessible for analysis. Without automatic data transfer, the task of entering data to be accessible to the command center may further burden the bedside staff.

The greatest barrier to implementation of tele-ICU is the cost. Evaluation of the capital investment versus the downstream financial benefit is available in the literature. Initial program development and the first year operational costs are estimated to between $50,000 and $100,000 per ICU bed when licensing software.[18,22] These costs were reduced to $21,967 for initial capital costs and $23,150 annual operational costs for a health system that built its own program, avoiding licensing fees associated with commercial products.[23] When placed in a cost-effectiveness analysis model where mortality benefit was assumed, a typical licensed tele-ICU was reported to be at least cost-effective and cost saving.[24] Subsets with cost benefits included those with a per-patient per-hospital-stay tele-ICU operation cost less than $1560, startup costs less than $851, or staffing and maintenance costs less than $1331 among other outlined parameters.[24] Cost figures incorporated into the model were estimated based on data from previously reported studies.[5,7,13,17,22,25,26]

A case study of a single academic center's journey with ICU telemedicine demonstrated financial benefits within their program that supported positive revenue.[27] The investigators outlined a timeline comparing a pre-ICU telemedicine period, a post-ICU telemedicine period, and a restructuring of the ICU telemedicine program to a logistic center. The logistic center managed team and bed assignments for all adult noncardiovascular critically ill patients through admission requests and discharging patients no longer critically ill. Quality care projects in numerous domains were implemented to support patient experience, patient care, and financial sustainability. Patient experience projects included efforts to keep the ICU quiet, and notification to and documentation of communication with primary care physicians, among others. The patient care redesign domain consisted of clinical practice guidelines, protocols, and standardized order sets for various conditions and complications that may be encountered in the ICU, such as pressure ulcers and tube feed placement.[27] Financial sustainability included guidelines for the use of high-cost medications and targeted processes to discharge patients to the floor or long-term acute care hospitals when able. Last, the integrated, safe, and high-quality care domain included projects aimed at preventing common iatrogenic ICU-related complications, such as venous-thromboembolism prophylaxis and catheter-associated urinary tract infections. Through the progression of this center's program, the benefits were twofold: a larger number of cases in the ICU secondary to decreased LOS and a larger revenue per case attributed to logistic center activities and quality-standardization and care-standardization projects. These findings are encouraging; however, they are limited to only a single academic center.

Hospital administrators place a value on the cost-effectiveness of tele-ICU implementation. Addition of services, such as new medications or devices, are supported by the developing manufacturers. Tele-ICU requires investment by health care organizations that implement them.[28] Organizations adopting a tele-ICU program may ensure cost-effectiveness by favoring systems for the highest-risk patients.[25,29] An observational study discovered that tele-ICU care was cost-effective for the sickest of patients with Simplified Acute Physiology II scores of greater than 50.[25] Similarly, Yoo and colleagues[29] developed a hypothetical tele-ICU model that resulted in cost-effectiveness in tertiary and community hospitals in both urban and rural settings when placing the 30% to 40% of the highest-risk patients as defined by their Acute Physiology and Chronic Health Evaluation IV score under monitoring.

Although barriers to implementation are inevitable, administrators in rural centers and academic centers should strongly consider these programs given their ability to address workforce shortages and provide cost-effective care.

WHERE DO WE GO NEXT?

Despite tele-ICU systems originating from a few vendors, variability in application of this technology exists. An updated survey of real-world tele-ICUs may identify best practices. Standardization and recommendations for essential components could follow. Additional efforts should focus to identify subsets of patients likely to benefit from a tele-ICU monitoring service. Critical care encompasses a wide range of conditions that affect various organ systems; however, intensivist monitoring may provide cost-effective care to improve outcomes in many different settings. Technology-based critical care systems have grown and continue to provide promise, there remains a need for hard outcome data with a focus on cost-effective targeted interventions to support widespread implementation.

REFERENCES

1. Fuhrman SA, Lilly CM. ICU telemedicine solutions. Clin Chest Med 2015;36(3): 401–7.
2. Angus DC, Shorr AF, White A, et al. Critical care delivery in the United States: distribution of services and compliance with Leapfrog recommendations. Crit Care Med 2006;34(4):1016–24.
3. The Leapfrog Group. Factsheet: ICU physician staffing. 2016. Available at: http://www.leapfroggroup.org/sites/default/files/Files/IPS Fact Sheet.pdf. Accessed October 10, 2017.
4. Castlight Health and The Leapfrog Group. Intensive care unit physician staffing: data by hospital on nationally standardized metrics. 2016. Available at: http://www.leapfroggroup.org/sites/default/files/Files/Castlight-Leapfrog-ICU-Physician-Staffing-Report-2016.pdf. Accessed October 10, 2017.
5. New England Healthcare Institute and Massachusettes Technology Collaborative. Critical care, critical choices: the case for tele-ICUs in intensive care. 2010. Available at: https://masstech.org/sites/mtc/files/documents/2010 TeleICU Report.pdf. Accessed October 10, 2017.
6. Reynolds HN, Rogove H, Bander J, et al. A working lexicon for the tele-intensive care unit: we need to define tele-intensive care unit to grow and understand it. Telemed J E Health 2011;17(10):773–83.
7. Lilly CM, McLaughlin JM, Zhao H, et al. A multicenter study of ICU telemedicine reengineering of adult critical care. Chest 2014;145(3):500–7.
8. Lilly CM, Fisher KA, Ries M, et al. A national ICU telemedicine survey: validation and results. Chest 2012;142(1):40–7.
9. Willmitch B, Golembeski S, Kim SS, et al. Clinical outcomes after telemedicine intensive care unit implementation. Crit Care Med 2012;40(2):450–4.
10. Morrison JL, Cai Q, Davis N, et al. Clinical and economic outcomes of the electronic intensive care unit: results from two community hospitals. Crit Care Med 2010;38(1):2–8.
11. McCambridge M, Jones K, Paxton H, et al. Association of health information technology and teleintensivist coverage with decreased mortality and ventilator use in critically ill patients. Arch Intern Med 2010;170(7):648–53.
12. Rosenfeld BA, Dorman T, Breslow MJ, et al. Intensive care unit telemedicine: alternate paradigm for providing continuous intensivist care. Crit Care Med 2000;28(12):3925–31.
13. Breslow MJ, Rosenfeld BA, Doerfler M, et al. Effect of a multiple-site intensive care unit telemedicine program on clinical and economic outcomes: an alternative paradigm for intensivist staffing. Crit Care Med 2004;32(1):31–8.

14. Nassar BS, Vaughan-Sarrazin MS, Jiang L, et al. Impact of an intensive care unit telemedicine program on patient outcomes in an integrated health care system. JAMA Intern Med 2014;174(7):1160.
15. Thomas EJ, Lucke JF, Wueste LR, et al. Association of telemedicine for remote monitoring of intensive care patients with mortality, complications, and length of stay. JAMA 2009;302(24):2671–8.
16. Wilcox ME, Adhikari NK. The effect of telemedicine in critically ill patients: systematic review and meta-analysis. Crit Care 2012;16(4):R127.
17. Young LB, Chan PS, Lu X, et al. Impact of telemedicine intensive care unit coverage on patient outcomes: a systematic review and meta-analysis. Arch Intern Med 2011;171(6):498–506.
18. Chen J, Sun D, Yang W, et al. Clinical and economic outcomes of telemedicine programs in the intensive care unit: a systematic review and meta-analysis. J Intensive Care Med 2017.
19. Kahn JM, Le TQ, Barnato AE, et al. ICU telemedicine and critical care mortality: a national effectiveness study. Med Care 2016;54(3):319–25.
20. Lilly CM, Cody S, Zhao H, et al. Hospital mortality, length of stay, and preventable complications among critically ill patients before and after tele-ICU reengineering of critical care processes. JAMA 2011;305(21):2175–83.
21. Berenson RA, Grossman JM, November EA. Does telemonitoring of patients–the eICU–improve intensive care? Health Aff 2009;28(5):w937–47.
22. Kumar G, Falk DM, Bonello RS, et al. The costs of critical care telemedicine programs: a systematic review and analysis. Chest 2013;143(1):19–29.
23. Fortis S, Weinert C, Bushinski R, et al. A health system-based critical care program with a novel tele-ICU: implementation, cost, and structure details. J Am Coll Surg 2014;219(4):676–83.
24. Yoo B-K, Kim M, Sasaki T, et al. Economic evaluation of telemedicine for patients in ICUs. Crit Care Med 2016;44(2):265–74.
25. Franzini L, Sail KR, Thomas EJ, et al. Costs and cost-effectiveness of a telemedicine intensive care unit program in 6 intensive care units in a large health care system. J Crit Care 2011;26(3):329.e1-6.
26. Cuthbertson BH, Roughton S, Jenkinson D, et al. Quality of life in the five years after intensive care: a cohort study. Crit Care 2010;14(1):R6.
27. Lilly CM, Motzkus C, Rincon T, et al. ICU telemedicine program financial outcomes. Chest 2017;151(2):286–97, e-Appendix 2.
28. Lilly CM, Motzkus CA. ICU telemedicine: financial analyses of a complex intervention. Crit Care Med 2017;45(9):1558–61.
29. Yoo B-K, Kim M, Sasaki T, et al. Selected use of telemedicine in intensive care units based on severity of illness improves cost-effectiveness. Telemed J E Health 2017;24(1):1–16.

Using Heuristic Evaluation to Improve Sepsis Alert Usability

Ariani Arista Putri Pertiwi, DNP, MSN, RN[a],
Dan Fraczkowski, MSN, RN[b], Sheryl L. Stogis, DrPH, RN[c],
Karen Dunn Lopez, PhD, MPH, RN[c],*

KEYWORDS

- Sepsis • Clinical decision support • Alerts • Early recognition • Usability
- Heuristic evaluation • Nursing informatics

KEY POINTS

- Sepsis alerts systems have been developed to help clinicians recognize and treat sepsis early to improve patient outcomes.
- Unfortunately, some alerts have poor usability and cause frustration that can compromise patient safety.
- Heuristic evaluation is a simple, easy to learn, and inexpensive systematic usability inspection method that can be used to identify problems in the usability of alert systems.
- Results from the heuristic evaluation can be delivered to the organization's health information technology and informatics leaders, as well as vendors, to improve the sepsis alert systems.

INTRODUCTION

Sepsis is an alarmingly common and life-threatening organ dysfunction caused by a dysregulated host response to infection.[1] Recent worldwide hospital mortality rates were 17% for sepsis and 26% for severe sepsis, with even higher rates in the United States.[2] It is the most expensive reason for hospital care,[3] with US hospitals spending

The authors have no commercial or financial conflicts of interests to report. Dr. A.A.P. Pertiwi was supported by a scholarship provided by the Directorate General of Resources for Science, Technology and Higher Education, Ministry of Research, Technology and Higher Education of Indonesia.
[a] Department of Basic Nursing and Emergency, Faculty of Medicine, Universitas Gadjah Mada, Jl, PSIK, FK, Farmako, Sekip Utara, Yogyakarta 55281, Indonesia; [b] Information Services, University of Illinois Hospital and Health Sciences System, 1740 W. Taylor Avenue, Chicago, IL 60612, USA; [c] Department of Health Systems Science, College of Nursing, University of Illinois at Chicago, 845 South Damen Avenue, Chicago, IL 60612, USA
* Corresponding author.
E-mail address: kdunnl2@uic.edu

over $ 55.6 million on sepsis care every day, and over $20 billion annually.[4] This problem is especially dire in intensive care units (ICUs), which care for the sickest patients in the hospital, where sepsis is the leading cause of death of critically ill patients cared for in non-coronary care ICUs.[5]

Early recognition of patients with sepsis is key to morbidity reduction,[6–9] reduced length of stay (LOS), cost per ICU stay,[10] and preventing sepsis mortality.[6,11–13] To improve sepsis care and outcomes, evidence-based guidelines have been widely disseminated.[14] The Society of Critical Care Medicine's Surviving Sepsis Campaign in particular has made great strides in improving awareness of sepsis, improving diagnosis, and developing guidelines.[15] They have also developed treatment bundles for both 3 hours and 6 hours from time of sepsis presentation (the earliest chart annotation with all elements of severe sepsis or septic shock ascertained through chart review)[16] to simplify the complexity of sepsis treatment. Despite these advances, the bundles do not eliminate complexity. The bundles require memory aides (such as printed badges) for the multiple steps and do not aide in early recognition. For these and other reasons, including epidemiologic causes such as increasing gram-positive organisms,[17] sepsis continues to be a major public health problem.

Clinical decision support (CDS) may overcome weaknesses in paper-based sepsis guidelines. CDS has been defined as "providing clinicians (nurses) with computer-generated clinical knowledge and patient related information which is intelligently filtered and presented at appropriate times to enhance patient care."[18] One factor of CDS includes clinical alarm systems that are intended to enhance safety by alerting clinicians to deviations from a predetermined normal status or potential patient problems.[18] Used within the electronic health record (EHR), CDS targeting clinician providers who direct care (eg, physicians and advanced practitioners) has been associated with improved process of care, reduced risk of morbidity, fewer medical errors, and increased compliance with standards of care.[19,20] More recently CDS has also been shown to improve patient outcomes when targeting decision making of bedside nurses.[21]

To better help both providers and bedside care nurses recognize sepsis as early as possible, several sepsis alerts systems have been developed. These sepsis CDS alerts reduce the need for external memory aides, streamline treatment ordering, and provide prompts for essential documentation. Designs of these alerts vary by: vendor, alert threshold trigger, and response required from providers to the alerts.[22,23]

The trigger thresholds for the alert system in this study are similar to the other sepsis alert systems identified in the literature. All are triggered by systemic inflammatory response syndrome (SIRS) criteria and at least one of organ dysfunction criteria. The alert system in this study used a higher heart rate trigger (>110 beats/minute, vs others that used >100 beats/minute). Although the published SIRS criteria is >90 beats/minute, the trigger was raised to decrease false-positive alert. Kurczewski and colleagues (2015) have the only other sepsis alert system the authors identified in the published literature.

In the alert reviewed in this study, registered nurses and medical doctors are required to respond to the alert that pops up in their patient's profile when they log in into the electronic health record by clicking the "OK" button. In contrast, Kurczewski and colleagues'[24] system provides a role-specific alert and response for each provider including care assistant, registered nurse, medical doctor, physician assistant, and nurse practitioner. For example, a care assistant can respond, "Will contact RN" or "RN Notified," while a medical doctor/physician assistant/nurse practitioner should select "Already Treating" or "Will Assess." Results after sepsis alert implementation are promising in Kurczewski and other studies, with statistically significant improvements in improved escalation of antibiotics and oxygen therapy[25] and reduced time to initial antibiotics and fluid resuscitation[25,26] and any sepsis-related intervention.[24]

Although CDS shows potential, as with all CDS alerts, if they are not properly designed or are difficult to use they lead to unintended consequences such as clinician frustration and can compromise patient safety.[27] When there is concern for these unintended consequences, it is reasonable to use formal methods to determine if the design and usability of the alert can be improved. This article reports on the application of a usability inspection method called heuristic evaluation of a sepsis alert system, designed by a major EHR vendor, in use in a tertiary hospital.

METHODS
Heuristic Evaluation

Heuristic evaluation is a systematic usability inspection method to identify and isolate problems as well as positive features in a user interface design.[28,29] This includes potential sources of confusion, unneeded complexity and steps, inconsistency, and navigation problems. Heuristic evaluation is most often used to identify technology design problems that impact usability and potential effectiveness before implementation. It is one of the usability methods that Nielsen coined as "discount usability engineering,"[30] meaning it does not require expensive laboratories and equipment, large staff, and contracted testers. The methodology can even be done without the evaluators interacting with a running system[30] using a paper prototype before a system is implemented. Detection of usability issues prior to implementation of a system can improve system performance and decrease the need for user support while reducing training costs. However, given the misconceptions and poor practices that many vendors have about rigorous user centered design,[28] the authors believe that heuristic evaluation can bring value to understanding ineffectiveness of electronic systems after implementation.

The authors used 14 usability principles[31] that have been used to explain a large proportion of problems with computer interfaces. The principles are largely based on the work of Nielsen's 10 rules[30] and Shneiderman's 8 golden rules of interface design.[32] Although other heuristics have been proposed, the advantage of the 14 usability principles the authors used is that they had already modified and applied for health care interfaces and specifically the EHR.[31] The principles included: consistency, visibility, match, minimalist, feedback, flexibility, error message, prevents errors, closure, undo, language, control, and help and documentation. General definitions of each principle and examples[33] are provided in **Table 1**.

Evaluators

Heuristic evaluation requires some background in usability and design to identify the full breadth of problems. However, the principles can be used by nonexperts as well to find many of the usability problems.[30] Three experts conducted the heuristic evaluation of the sepsis alert system for this project. As recommended by Georgsson, the authors used dual domain experts[34]; two in usability, clinical decision support, informatics, and health care and one who also had expertise with the hospital's EHR system.

Rating Scale

The authors adapted the 5-level rating scale,[35] based on the severity level of the usability problem. Zero indicated no usability problem; 1 = cosmetic problems that modifying may improve clinicians' satisfaction; 2 = minor usability problem that may cause clinicians' confusion, and 3 = major usability problems that can

Table 1
Heuristic principles

Principles	Definition
Consistency	The design features should appear uniformly and have consistent meaning throughout the system.
Visibility	Users should be informed regarding what is going on with the system
Match	Match between the system and the world; it matches the common meaning outside the system
Minimalist	Minimalist at the design, as necessary toward the objectives of the system
Memory	The system provides cues for user doing data input when needed. For example, the pattern MM/DD/YY for month, date, and year
Feedback	Informative information should be provided as feedback by the system to end users about their actions
Flexibility	Shortcuts such as function keys or command keys allow flexibility of use for frequently used operations
Error Message	Messages should provide adequate, timely information to allow for action and error recovery
Prevent Error	Prevent users from making mistakes; is the system designed to prevent errors and/or mitigate errors if they occur?
Closure	Every task has a beginning and an end; users should be clearly notified when a task has been completed
Undo	Reversible actions. Human error should be anticipated, and the user is given the opportunity to recover from slips, lapses and mistakes.
Language	The language should be presented in a form understandable by the intended users.
Control	The user should be able to understand how to navigate the EHR with ease.
Help and documentation	If the users require assistance, how would they obtain it? Avoid reliance on user manuals at the point of care. Embedded help is preferred.

compromise patient safety. The fifth level, usability catastrophe that is imperative to fix before implementation was not identified in this alert.

Scenario

The authors focused their evaluation on the 2 major components of the sepsis alert interface: the pop-up alert window and the complete sepsis alert workflow. The alert window appears on the EHR interface when the patient has at least 2 characteristics of the following signs and symptoms: respiratory rate of more than 24 times per minute, heart rate more than 110 beats per minute (bpm), temperature of more than 38° C or less than 36° C, white blood cells count of more than 12,000 cells/mm^3 or less than 4000 cells/mm^3, plasma glucose more than 140 mg/dL in patients without diabetes. Additionally, at least of the following organ dysfunction signs should be present: systolic blood pressure (SBP) less than 90 mm Hg or mean arterial pressure (MAP) less than 65 mm Hg, lactate more than 2.0 mmol/L, creatinine increase from the baseline 0.5 mg/dL, and bilirubin of 2.0 mg/dL up to 10.0 mg/dL (Personal Communication, Institution's Department of Nursing). The complete sepsis alert workflow includes nurses and physicians' tasks: acknowledging the alert, sepsis bundle treatment activation, and documentation.

Procedures

As part of the evaluation process, the team met to review and develop a common understanding of each of the 14 heuristics. Using multiple sources,[32,33,35] the authors then developed an evaluation scoring tool (Appendix 1) with each principle, definitions, and examples. Subsequently, 2 evaluators independently reviewed interface components using a test patient alert. This was an interactive training alert created by the hospital's information technology department using fictitious patient data. Once data were entered that matched the sepsis criteria, the sepsis alert window appeared as expected.

Scoring data were collected on a spreadsheet denoting the heuristic principles violated for each component of the interface, the score of severity, and the expert rationale of giving the score. Once each expert completed his or her evaluation, the heuristic violations were aggregated into a single list to compare evaluation agreement and disagreement. The third expert, a doctorally prepared usability, clinical decision support, and informatics expert, met with the 2 evaluators to discuss disagreement and develop consensus on the usability problems and severity of all 14 heuristic principles. This includes usability problems that violated more than one heuristic. When violation of a heuristic principle could have more than 1 outcome (eg, could compromise safety and cause confusion), the authors scored the highest severity (=3).

Results

Experts identified usability flaws in the 12 of 14 heuristic principles across the sepsis alert workflow for a total of 21 specific usability problems uncovered. **Table 2** shows the complete list of violations on heuristic principles and its severity that the authors observed in the system. They found 4 violations on the heuristic principle of consistency: 3 violations on the principle of visibility (severity score = 2); 2 violations on the principles of match (severity score = 3 and 2); minimalism (severity score = 2); flexibility (severity score = 2); prevent error (severity score = 3); 1 violation in each of the principles of feedback (score = 3); *message* (score = 2); undo (score = 3); language (score = 2); control (score = 2) and documentation (score = 2). Severity scores ranged from 1 to 3; 28% were classified as major usability problems (score = 3), and 52% met criteria as minor usability problems (score = 2). The remaining 20% were cosmetic problems (score = 1).

The consistency principle means that the design features should appear uniformly and have consistent meaning throughout the system.[37] This includes the colors and icons used. For example, the authors found that colors were used to convey different meaning in the interface. In 1 part of the interface (medication order set), green and blue are used to differentiate medication options based on the sepsis sources. However, the green and blue colors are not used in other locations in the interface. In another violation of the consistency principle, the authors found 2o different cross buttons appeared in the same interface (**Fig. 1**), causing confusion. One of the cross-buttons, if erroneously selected, eliminates the sepsis notification. As a result, clinicians may acknowledge the alert but not be able to review which patient presented with sepsis signs and symptoms. Another violation of consistency is the different font type and size in the pop-up window. This resulted in too much information displayed and may have decreased the sense of urgency to act upon the alert.

Visibility means that the users should be provided feedback regarding what the system is processing. For example, the alert did not have information provided to tell clinicians that the orders they input are being processed, which can lead to attempts to duplicate order entry. Also, the information displayed on the pop-up

Table 2
Observed heuristic violations

Heuristic Principles	Observed Violations	Score
Consistency	Although colors draw attention to order specific set of medication for specific sepsis source, the colors are not used in other locations in the system, which may confuse clinicians might take time to figure out what does that mean.	1
	Two different sign buttons appear in the order screen.	1
	Two different red cross buttons appear in overdue discern alerts which caused clinicians' confusion.	3
	Different font type and size in the initial discern alert.	1
Visibility	No information is available from the system to tell providers that orders are being processed, which leads to confusion, especially for new providers.	2
	Information alerting the clinician of potential sepsis which is could be larger and in a more visual shape. Parameters that triggered the alert could be displayed in bulleted form.	2
	The alert window is not large enough to contain all relevant information when it initially appears, requiring the user to stretch the window to fit.	2
Match	Icons (4 icons) have no easily discernible meaning. Hovering over the icon will give the user information about the icon meaning. User might document in the wrong location. Essential information is difficult to locate by other team member which may lead to inaccurate documentation because the user put in the wrong time line.	3
	An Icon available to close the alert is shaped as folder and arrow. Some icons provided are not active.	2
Minimalism	A number "80" appears in the initial sepsis alert that has no meaning related to patient care	2
	There are 6 patient identifications take spaces for other information to be displayed.	1
Memory	No violation observed	0
Feedback	No prompt messages appear before clinicians click the 'x' button that will erase the alert message forever.	3
Flexibility	The search field does not function, as a clinician would expect in the standard. In order to locate a provider for notification, the nurse must type in the complete provider name and then select a Magnifying glass icon, then click enter to execute the search	2
	There is no shortcut or clickable link to bring clinicians to required action/intervention pages.	2
Message	The error message does not direct the user to the recommended action.	2
Prevent error	The initial alert can't be minimized, but it can be deleted. Clinicians may forget the alert once it is deleted prior to addressing it.	3
	The time stamp for documentation defaults to the time the alert was fired, with no prompt for the user to adjust time when they document the intervention. This may lead to inaccurate documentation.	3
Closure	No violation observed	0

(continued on next page)

Table 2
(continued)

Heuristic Principles	Observed Violations	Score
Undo	Once the initial alert is closed, there is no way to retrieve it again. This may lead to patient harm	3
Language	The word "Discern Alert" is not a familiar term for clinicians.	2
Control	There is no clear instruction on what actions the nurse needs to take. Novice nurses and floating nurses might confuse what actions are necessary. Clicking "X" in the alert is expected to bring the clinician to the intervention page interface.	2
Documentation	The alert provides lots of information, but it is not task oriented. There is no easily accessible help section	2

window is too cluttered, and the window itself is too small when it appears, requiring the clinicians to stretch it out to make it bigger so that they can see all information of the alert.

The match principle refers to match in meaning between the system and the common meaning in the real world (eg, the common meaning of red is stop). **Fig. 2** displays icon symbols where the meanings were not discernible to any of the 3 experts.

The feedback principle refers to information that should be provided as feedback by the system to end users about their actions. For example, there were no immediate

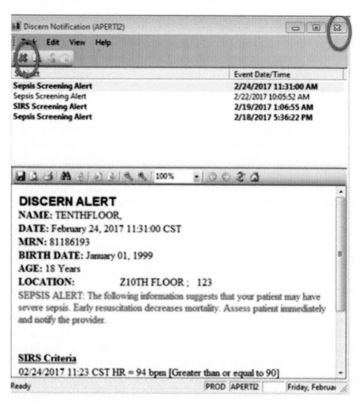

Fig. 1. Two different cross-buttons appeared in the same interface.

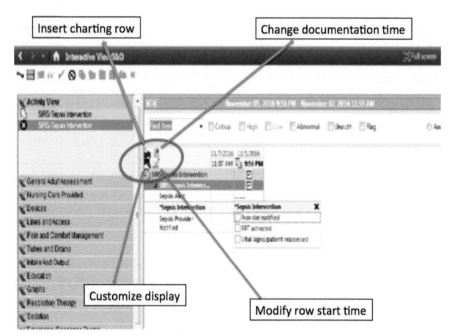

Fig. 2. Icon symbols where the meanings were not discernible to any of the 3 experts.

messages that appeared to inform the clinician that pressing the X button would forever erase the information about patients who met the sepsis criteria. This creates the potential for clinicians to forget which patient met sepsis criteria and needed timely treatment.

DISCUSSION

The various manifestations of sepsis can be difficult to detect. Although sepsis alerts intend to improve early recognition and treatment, results of this project indicate the need for improving the usability of the sepsis alert system being evaluated. Similar to other heuristic evaluations,[29,33,34,36–39] the authors found many usability problems. Thankfully, in this postimplementation study, the authors did not identify any catastrophic problems. Nonetheless, they found many problems that can cause patient safety problems, such as deleting patients.

The most common problems in the sepsis alert system the authors evaluated were the usability violations in the principles of consistency, match, feedback, prevent error, and undo. All of these violations have the potential to harm patients. The authors also found many design problems that can cause confusion for clinicians. Confusion may sound minor; however, confusion can cause frustration, decrease work efficiency, and increase cognitive load.

Issues in match between the real world and the alert design are illustrated by the bar graph icon. Many people may interpret a bar graph icon in the way bar graphs are used in the real world, as a feature to make a graph from the data recorded in the system. However, in this particular interface, the bar graph icon is used to insert new charting raw by the time when the clinicians record the data. Because it does not match the real-world use of making a graph, places additional cognitive demands on the user to use his or her memory that the bar graph was the symbol for inserting new charting raw (see **Fig. 2**). Further, another icon appears to contain a graph and eraser that allows the user to customize the flow sheet display, when in the real world (and other interfaces), erase icons are used to erase text or data. These icons are used across the sepsis alert flow sheet documentation, and despite hover-over functionality that causes explanatory text to appear about the function, the mismatch to the user's expectation of what the icon should be can cause unnecessary confusion.

Consistent with the heuristic evaluation method, the authors did not include the views of actual clinician users.[30] This step is important and can be done in conjunction with or to validate or broaden findings of the heuristic evaluation. However, many usability heuristic violations may be outside of the awareness of clinicians.[38] Therefore problems identified by experts as violating known design heuristics should be addressed even if clinicians do not recognize them as a problem.

Heuristic evaluation is a feasible usability testing method that provides an easy, quick, and inexpensive usability testing for a graphical user interface. Heuristic evaluation as an expert-based usability testing method[40] is only one among several usability tools that can be used, and it may benefit from additional heuristics to improve usability of clinical technologies.[40,41] User feedback as a user-based method, user-centered design[40] and observations of use in practice are also important to get a comprehensive result of usability testing.

LIMITATION

One limitation of a heuristic evaluation is the subjectivity of the experts. The author used 3 strategies to minimize subjectivity: (1) use of multiple evaluators, (2) a heuristic evaluation scoring tool that included definition of each principles and a situation example, and (3) synchronous consensus sessions after independent scoring to thoroughly discuss any disagreements. In addition, heuristic evaluation does not include additional perceptions that users may detect that are not obvious to expert reviewers. Thus, the process of evaluating usability in health care technologies must also use other methods to include the perceptions of clinical users.

SUMMARY

Sepsis alert systems are being used frequently in health care, but many of them have usability problems. Heuristic evaluation is a simple and inexpensive usability testing that can uncover usability issues of these alert systems. This is particularly important to sepsis alert systems, because a more usable alert may improve clinicians' ability to detect and act upon the alerts, which in turn can decrease sepsis related mortality. Clinicians should be familiar with what heuristic principles are. Knowing these principles gives clinicians who may have a hunch of why something is frustrating the vocabulary to convey the possible reasons to their organization leaders and vendor liaison. Disseminating heuristic evaluation knowledge to clinicians and developing training programs related to heuristic principles for clinicians could extend the impact of this method and lead to improvements in CDS systems and EHR's usability.

REFERENCES

1. Singer M, Deutschman CS, Seymour CW, et al. The third international consensus definitions for sepsis and septic shock (sepsis-3). JAMA 2016;315(8):801–10.
2. Fleischmann C, Scherag A, Adhikari NK, et al. Assessment of global incidence and mortality of hospital-treated sepsis. Current estimates and limitations. Am J Respir Crit Care Med 2016;193(3):259–72.

3. O'Brien J. The cost of sepsis. 2015. Available at: https://blogs.cdc.gov/safehealthcare/the-cost-of-sepsis/. Accessed September 25, 2017.
4. Pfuntner A, Wier LM, Steiner C. Costs for hospital stays in the United States, 2011: statistical brief# 168. Agency for Healthcare Research and Quality; 2006.
5. Angus DC, Linde-Zwirble WT, Lidicker J, et al. Epidemiology of severe sepsis in the United States: analysis of incidence, outcome, and associated costs of care. Crit Care Med 2001;29(7):1303–10.
6. Jones SL, Ashton CM, Kiehne L, et al. Reductions in sepsis mortality and costs after design and implementation of a nurse-based early recognition and response program. Jt Comm J Qual Patient Saf 2015;41(11):483–91.
7. Ramar K, Gajic O. Early recognition and treatment of severe sepsis. Am J Respir Crit Care Med 2013;188:7–8.
8. Umscheid CA, Betesh J, VanZandbergen C, et al. Development, implementation, and impact of an automated early warning and response system for sepsis. J Hosp Med 2015;10(1):26–31.
9. Westphal GA, Lino AS. Systematic screening is essential for early diagnosis of severe sepsis and septic shock. Rev Bras Ter Intensiva 2015;27(2):96–101.
10. Judd WR, Stephens DM, Kennedy CA. Clinical and economic impact of a quality improvement initiative to enhance early recognition and treatment of sepsis. Ann Pharmacother 2014;48(10):1269–75.
11. Soong J, Soni N. Sepsis: recognition and treatment. Clin Med 2012;12(3):276–80.
12. Sterling SA, Miller WR, Pryor J, et al. The impact of timing of antibiotics on outcomes in severe sepsis and septic shock: a systematic review and meta-analysis. Crit Care Med 2015;43(9):1907.
13. Lilly CM. The ProCESS trial–a new era of sepsis management. N Engl J Med 2014;370(18):1750.
14. Rhodes A, Evans LE, Alhazzani W, et al. Surviving sepsis campaign: international guidelines for management of sepsis and septic shock: 2016. Intensive Care Med 2017;43(3):304–77.
15. Surviving Sepsis Campaign Guidelines. 2016. Available at: http://www.survivingsepsis.org/Guidelines/Pages/default.aspx. Accessed September 25, 2017.
16. Surviving Sepsis Campaign. Updated bundles in response to new evidence 2016. http://www.survivingsepsis.org/SiteCollectionDocuments/SSC_Bundle.pdf. Accessed September 25, 2017.
17. Mayr FB, Yende S, Angus DC. Epidemiology of severe sepsis. Virulence 2014;5(1):4–11.
18. Teich JM, Osheroff JA, Pifer EA, et al. Clinical decision support in electronic prescribing: recommendations and an action plan: report of the joint clinical decision support workgroup. J Am Med Inform Assoc 2005;12(4):365–76.
19. Bright TJ, Wong A, Dhurjati R, et al. Effect of clinical decision-support systemsa systematic review. Ann Intern Med 2012;157(1):29–43.
20. Sidebottom AC, Collins B, Winden TJ, et al. Reactions of nurses to the use of electronic health record alert features in an inpatient setting. Comput Inform Nurs 2012;30(4):218–26.
21. Dunn Lopez K, Gephart SM, Raszewski R, et al. Integrative review of clinical decision support for registered nurses in acute care settings. J Am Med Inform Assoc 2017;24(2):441–50.
22. Makam AN, Nguyen OK, Auerbach AD. Diagnostic accuracy and effectiveness of automated electronic sepsis alert systems: a systematic review. J Hosp Med 2015;10(6):396–402.

23. Miliard M. With EHR-based sepsis detection, epic and cerner have different approaches. 2017. Available at: http://www.healthcareitnews.com/news/ehr-based-sepsis-detection-epic-and-cerner-have-different-approaches. Accessed October 19, 2017.

24. Kurczewski L, Sweet M, McKnight R, et al. Reduction in time to first action as a result of electronic alerts for early sepsis recognition. Crit Care Nurs Q 2015;38(2):182–7.

25. Sawyer AM, Deal EN, Labelle AJ, et al. Implementation of a real-time computerized sepsis alert in nonintensive care unit patients. Crit Care Med 2011;39(3):469–73.

26. Hayden GE, Tuuri RE, Scott R, et al. Triage sepsis alert and sepsis protocol lower times to fluids and antibiotics in the ED. Am J Emerg Med 2016;34(1):1–9.

27. Guardia-LaBar LM, Scruth EA, Edworthy J, et al. Alarm fatigue: the human-system interface. Clin Nurse Spec 2014;28(3):135–7.

28. Ratwani RM, Fairbanks RJ, Hettinger AZ, et al. Electronic health record usability: analysis of the user-centered design processes of eleven electronic health record vendors. J Am Med Inform Assoc 2015;22(6):1179–82.

29. Reolon M, Lacerda TC, Krone C, et al. Usability heuristics for evaluating health-care applications for smartphones: a systematic literature review. 2016. Available at: https://www.researchgate.net/profile/Aldo_Von_Wangenheim2/publication/313009902_Usability_Heuristics_for_Evaluating_Health_care_Applications_for_Smartphones_A_Systematic_Literature_Review/links/588c53f8aca272fa50df1dcb/Usability-Heuristics-for-Evaluating-Health-care-Applications-for-Smartphones-A-Systematic-Literature-Review.pdf

30. Nielsen J. Usability engineering. San Diego (CA): Elsevier; 1994.

31. Zhang J, Walji MF. TURF: toward a unified framework of EHR usability. J Biomed Inform 2011;44(6):1056–67.

32. Shneiderman B. Designing for fun: how can we design user interfaces to be more fun? Interactions 2004;11(5):48–50.

33. Harrington L, Porch L, Acosta K, et al. Realizing electronic medical record benefits: an easy-to-do usability study. J Nurs Adm 2011;41(7–8):331–5.

34. Georgsson M, Staggers N, Weir C. A modified user-oriented heuristic evaluation of a mobile health system for diabetes self-management support. Comput Inform Nurs 2016;34(2):77.

35. Nielsen J. Severity ratings for usability problems. 1995. Available at: https://www.nngroup.com/articles/how-to-rate-the-severity-of-usability-problems/. Accessed December 2, 2016, 2016.

36. Zhang J, Johnson TR, Patel VL, et al. Using usability heuristics to evaluate patient safety of medical devices. J Biomed Inform 2003;36(1):23–30.

37. Schnall R, Bakken S, Brown W III, et al. Usabilty evaluation of a prototype mobile App for health management for persons living with HIV. Stud Health Technol Inform 2016;225:481.

38. LeRouge C, Hasselquist MB, Kellogg L, et al. Using heuristic evaluation to enhance the visual display of a provider dashboard for patient-reported outcomes. eGEMs (Generating Evidence & Methods to improve patient outcomes) 2017;5(2):1–12.

39. Preece MH, Hill A, Horswill MS, et al. Applying heuristic evaluation to observation chart design to improve the detection of patient deterioration. Appl Ergon 2013;44(4):544–56.

40. Jaspers MW. A comparison of usability methods for testing interactive health technologies: methodological aspects and empirical evidence. Int J Med Inform 2009;78(5):340–53.

41. Sousa VE, Lopez KD. Towards usable e-health. Appl Clin Inform 2017;8(2):470–90.

APPENDIX 1: HEURISTIC EVALUATION TOOL

Scale
- 0 = No problems
- 1 = Cosmetic problem
- 2 = Minor usability problem
- 3 = Major usability problem: high priority to fix
- 4 = Usability catastrophe

Heuristic	Scale 0 1 2 3 4	Rationale
Consistency		
This includes consistency in the use of font, spacing, layout, and color		
Visibility		
Features within the EHR that display what the system is processing (eg, a spinning circle that communicates information is downloading)		
Match		
This applies to how icons and symbols that are used in the system match how it is used in the real world (eg, use of a red octagon can effectively cue the need to stop an action)		
Minimalist		
Interface displays that do not contain any irrelevant or extra information and contain ample white space to decrease the appearance of being cluttered		
Minimize memory load		
This can include cues for how to input data such as MM/DD/YY and use of a common icon such as a magnifying glass for searching		
Informative feedback		
This includes information provided to the clinicians that is helpful to clinicians using the EHR (eg, a text box that displays the words: "SUBMITTED CORRECTLY" after correct submissions)		
Flexibility		
The availability for shortcuts that allow expert users to navigate and use quickly		
Messages		
This includes messages that provide understandable information to the clinician (eg, error code #K123 does not tell the clinician what the cause of the error is and what to do next)		
Prevent errors		
Examples include not permitting: 4 digits to be entered for systolic blood pressure or a message that displays "ARE YOU SURE YOU WANT TO DELETE THIS?" before deleting		
Closure		
An example would be a "COMPLETE" message that displays when task is complete		

(continued on next page)

(continued)

Heuristic	Scale					Rationale
	0	1	2	3	4	
Undo						
Easy-to-find opportunities to undo data entry that clinicians notice they input incorrectly						
Language						
Use of everyday language that is consistent with the meaning of it in the real world (eg, the heading "PHYSICAL EXAM "is more easily understood than "ENCOUNTER PHYSICAL DATA")						
Control						
The clinician should be able to understand ways to controlling the system						
Help and Documentation						
Strong EHR design should prevent the need for routine help; however, help feature should be available, easy to find and understand						

Courtesy of Ariani Arista Putri Pertiwi, DNP, MAN, RN, Yogyakarta, Indonesia and Karen Dunn Lopez, PhD, MPH, RN, Chicago, IL.

Printed and bound by CPI Group (UK) Ltd, Croydon, CR0 4YY

07/10/2024

01040500-0011